CRISIS AND CARE
QUEER ACTIVIST RESPONSES TO A GLOBAL PANDEMIC

Edited by Adrian Shanker
Foreword by Rea Carey

Crisis and Care: Queer Activist Responses to a Global Pandemic
Adrian Shanker © 2022
This edition © PM Press

ISBN: 978-1-62963-935-2 (paperback)
ISBN: 978-1-62963-949-9 (ebook)
Library of Congress Control Number: 2021945067

Cover design by John Yates/www.stealworks.com
Interior design by briandesign

10 9 8 7 6 5 4 3 2 1

PM Press
PO Box 23912
Oakland, CA 94623
www.pmpress.org

Printed in the USA

For my grandmother
Eadie Gerber Shanker
who never stopped fighting for what she believed in.

May her memory be a blessing.

"Only by mourning everything we have lost
can we discover that we have in fact survived;
that our spirits are indestructible."
—Aurora Levins Morales

CONTENTS

FOREWORD

Rea Carey

Over the course of my thirty years in the LGBTQ+ movement, including seventeen years at the National LGBTQ Task Force, I have seen our LGBTQ+ movement adapt to trying times before. We have shown up for each other. But the sudden and significant changes to our lives because of the COVID-19 pandemic were different—it wasn't anything like what we had experienced before. It immediately surfaced and magnified existing health access disparities, as well as discrimination, especially for Black and Brown members of our community and for trans and gender nonconforming people. Yet the LGBTQ+ community quickly created virtual connections, assessed the immediate impact, launched mutual aid efforts, modeled resiliency, and demanded health equity. The LGBTQ+ community responded to a global pandemic with determination that we would all get through it together, and that the most vulnerable members of our community would have our collective support—and, importantly, that we had much to teach the rest of the country about responding to a health crisis being mishandled by the government, as was the case during the early years of HIV/ AIDS.

Like all of us, the LGBTQ+ movement didn't have a roadmap for navigating COVID-19, but we worked to figure it out together. This book presents a collection of essays that demonstrate how our community responded. We should remember this moment in time. We should always respond with the care and resiliency that our LGBTQ+ movement demonstrated throughout this crisis. No doubt we will need that strength again.

INTRODUCTION
Adrian Shanker

All of a sudden, the world stopped. Or at least it felt that way. Airports were empty, public schools closed, colleges sent their students home. The media even reported that the COVID-19 shutdown led to a drastic reduction in air pollution, leading to "alpine weather" in the crowded city of Delhi. Quite literally, nothing felt normal. We started to hear from friends that someone they knew was sick, or that someone they knew had died. We heard from many more that they were out of work, or worse: required to work without personal protective equipment to keep themselves safe. In this moment, everything that seemed impossible became our reality.

These were dark times, but when it's dark out, there is an opportunity to shine a light, and that's what this book is about.

This is not a book exploring the infectiousness of a novel coronavirus or recounting experiences for the archives. Many others will write or edit those books. This is a book about queer activism and resiliency during a global pandemic. It is about what we learned from a seminal moment in our lives and how we will utilize these lessons to inform our activism in the future. We will explore how queer people advocated, insisted, and demanded that our health and economic needs be met. We will explore how queer people held each other and cared for each other and modeled resiliency for the whole world to see. We will explore how queer activists responded to a global pandemic.

The COVID-19 pandemic was not a fleeting moment in time. It was a time that anyone who lived through it will remember for the rest of their life. Our lives were traumatically disrupted, with any semblance of normalcy gone. Queer activists made hand-sewn masks to keep their communities safe. Queer activists created mutual aid programs to meet the urgent needs of the most marginalized members of our community. Queer activists used technology to create virtual connections many of us didn't know existed before. Queer activists demanded that the broken health care system respond to queer community needs. Queer activists asked pointed questions. We demanded that our government prioritize people over profits. We demanded that workers be treated as heroes. We advocated for the abolition of prisons, perhaps especially when they resembled petri dishes likely to spread a dangerous virus. We demanded data collection about our community's unique vulnerability to COVID-19. We demanded information about how to safely have sex during a pandemic, and when information wasn't available, queer people created the information ourselves.

In short, activism, community care, and resiliency saved us from loneliness, boredom, and desperation. The urgency of every fight was motivation to get out of bed the next day. The determination to hold our community close, even from afar, meant that we could find new ways to care for each other. LGBTQ+ people were clear that this was not our first virus, that we as a population knew something about how to survive a plague. Queer people were not the ones demanding that businesses reopen before it was safe. Queer people were not the ones questioning why we should wear face masks or protesting vaccine mandates. Queer people were not the ones trying to put profit before people. Queer activists responded to COVID-19 with love, care, and community. Queer activists responded with hope and resiliency. Poet and activist Grace Paley once said, "Let us go forth with fear and courage and rage," and that's exactly the combination of feelings we held in our hearts. Scholars will be writing and retelling the stories from the COVID-19 pandemic for years. The lessons we learned in the first half of 2020 are lessons that will inform our activism for years to come. Just as this was not our first virus, it also is unlikely to be our last. The intention of this book is to consider these lessons, so we can collectively apply them as we prepare our communities and our world for the crisis points we will encounter next.

Living through a pandemic is a traumatic experience. This book seeks to lift up queer responses to COVID-19. Queer people responded to a crisis with care, and by doing so lived out Paley's directive of going forth with fear, courage, and rage. All that we had was each other. Luckily, it turns out that this was all that we needed.

ELIMINATING HEALTH CARE DISCRIMINATION DURING A PUBLIC HEALTH CRISIS

Jamie Gliksberg and Omar Gonzalez-Pagan

The COVID-19 pandemic markedly changed our lives in 2020. In the span of five months, more than two million Americans tested positive, and over one hundred thousand Americans died in less than four months.[1] The public health crisis that ensued showed in particularly stark terms why access to health care is essential for every person and why we need to foster trust between health care providers and the public.

Unfortunately, LGBTQ+ people, like many other minorities, face systemic and pervasive discrimination in many aspects of life. This includes, quite dangerously, the realm of health care. Oftentimes, when accessing health care, LGBTQ+ people encounter disparate treatment and lack of coverage. Statements like "we don't provide services to *people like you*" and "your *kind* needs to go elsewhere" are tragically familiar to LGBTQ+ people.

In this short essay, we focus on three points. First, the lived experiences of LGBTQ+ people and their families, which demonstrate why protections from discrimination are necessary in health care. Second, how existing protections rooted in state law and, most particularly, the Affordable Care Act (ACA), enacted in 2010, have helped remedy some of the discrimination faced by LGBTQ+ people. However, these protections are under attack and we must ensure their expansion, not their diminishment. Last, we discuss, based on our experience as movement lawyers, how litigation efforts that represent

LGBTQ+ organizations and LGBTQ+-affirming health care providers can help protect our victories and turn away the misguided attacks on LGBTQ+ people's access to health care.

Why We Need LGBTQ+ Health Care Protections

There are approximately thirteen to fourteen million LGBTQ+ people in the United States.[2] Yet discrimination against LGBTQ+ and gender nonconforming people in health care is rampant. LGBTQ+ and gender nonconforming people routinely report: being refused needed care; health care professionals refusing to touch them or using excessive precautions; health care professionals using harsh or abusive language; being blamed for their health status; and health care professionals being physically rough or abusive.

In 2010, Lambda Legal published a study focused on the experiences of LGBTQ+ people with health care. The study, *When Health Care Isn't Caring*, showed that almost 56 percent of LGB people and 70 percent of transgender and gender nonconforming people have had one or more of the aforementioned discriminatory experiences.[3] In fact, 8 percent of LGB people and 27 percent of transgender and gender nonconforming people have been denied health care altogether.

Subsequent studies have further documented these experiences. A 2017 study by the Center for American Progress similarly showed that LGBTQ+ people face disturbing rates of health care discrimination: from harassment and humiliation by providers to being turned away by hospitals, pharmacists, and doctors.[4] According to the 2017 study, 8 percent of LGBQ respondents stated that a doctor or other health care provider refused to see them because of their actual or perceived sexual orientation, and 6 percent said that a doctor or other health care provider refused to give them health care related to their actual or perceived sexual orientation. The numbers, once again, were even more alarming for transgender people, as 29 percent of transgender respondents said a doctor or other health care provider refused to see them because of their actual or perceived gender identity, 23 percent said a doctor or other health care provider intentionally misgendered them or used the wrong name, and 21 percent said a doctor or other health care provider used harsh or abusive language when treating them.

Similarly, the 2015 US Transgender Survey, a study that surveyed 27,715 transgender and gender nonconforming individuals, showed that one-third of transgender people who had seen a health care provider reported having at least one negative experience related to being transgender, such as verbal harassment, refusal of treatment, or having to teach the health care provider about transgender people to receive appropriate care.[5] In addition, more than half of transgender people who sought coverage for gender-affirming health care were denied. More specifically, one in four of those who sought coverage for hormones and 55 percent of those who sought coverage for gender-affirming surgery were denied coverage.

These numbers are even more stark when one looks at the experiences of LGBTQ+ people of color, older adults, and youth who are homeless or in the custody of the state.[6]

These glaring numbers demonstrate why LGBTQ+ people need protections from discrimination in health care. They are key to ensuring their health and well-being. These experiences also show why these protections from discrimination in health care are necessary to ensure the health and well-being of every person, particularly in times of a public health crisis. That is because negative experiences in health care serve as a deterrent for people seeking medical care. They cement distrust and a lack of confidence.

The 2017 Center for American Progress study showed that discrimination played a role in preventing a significant number of LGBTQ+ people from seeking health care. For example, in the year prior to the survey, 8 percent of all LGBTQ+ people and 14 percent of those who had experienced discrimination on the basis of their sexual orientation or gender identity in the past year avoided or postponed needed medical care because of disrespect or discrimination from health care staff. Among transgender people, 22 percent reported such avoidance. The 2015 US Transgender Survey backs up these numbers. This survey indicated that 23 percent of respondents did not see a doctor when they needed to because of fear of being mistreated as a transgender person.

These numbers represent a serious public health problem, because a lack of timely access to prevention and treatment services results in poorer health outcomes and added costs.[7] It also prevents people from seeking care in times of crisis, which is pivotal to responding to a pandemic. As our experience with COVID-19 illustrates, testing and contact tracing are key elements to any effective response to a pandemic.[8]

Existing LGBTQ+ Protections from Discrimination in Health Care

We have made significant progress in enacting protections from discrimination in state and federal law over the last few years. For example, as of June 2020, 37 percent of LGBTQ+ people live in states with insurance protections that include sexual orientation and gender identity,[9] and 49 percent of LGBTQ+ people live in states that explicitly prohibit discrimination in public accommodations based on sexual orientation and gender identity.[10] In addition, the Affordable Care Act, enacted in 2010, includes a provision known as Section 1557 that prohibits discrimination on the basis of sex in health care programs and activities that receive federal funding.[11] Consistent with the interpretation by a majority of federal courts, in 2016, the United States Department of Health and Human Services (HHS) interpreted this prohibition to encompass discrimination based on gender identity and sex stereotypes following years of federal rulemaking.[12]

While there is much work yet to be done, the Affordable Care Act's Section 1557 has proven crucial to eliminating health disparities for LGBTQ+ people. Indeed, a study by the Center for American Progress analyzing complaints of discrimination based on gender identity, sexual orientation, and sexual orientation–related sex stereotyping that were investigated and closed by HHS's Office of Civil Rights between March 2010 and January 2017 showed that the enforcement of the ACA's Section 1557 was working well to resolve very real issues of discrimination.[13]

As LGBTQ+ rights advocates, we have seen firsthand how these protections have been effective at remedying discrimination against LGBTQ+ people. Indeed, Section 1557 has proven critical to eliminating discriminatory exclusions of coverage for gender-affirming care,[14] as well as remedying discriminatory treatment of LGBTQ+ people by health care providers and staff.[15]

Protections from Discrimination Were Under Attack

Notwithstanding the clear need for protections from discrimination for LGBTQ+ people and the demonstrated effectiveness of these protections, anti-LGBTQ+ activists and the Trump administration sought to undermine these protections. As a result, considerable efforts and resources were dedicated to defending these critical protections from attack.

For example, in May 2019, HHS, under the Trump administration, announced the promulgation of a new rule that invited discrimination against LGBTQ+ people in health care by purporting to create broad rights to empower health care providers and staff to deny health care treatment to LGBTQ+ people based on the providers' religious or moral beliefs.[16] In response, Lambda Legal, in conjunction with the Center for Reproductive Rights, Americans United for Separation of Church and State, and pro bono counsel at Mayer Brown, coordinating with the County of Santa Clara, filed a lawsuit weeks later challenging the legality of the rule.[17] We discuss this lawsuit in greater detail below, but suffice it to say that we successfully stopped it from taking effect, at least as of the time of this essay.[18]

Later in 2019, HHS announced that it would stop enforcing antidiscrimination protections, including protections based on gender identity or sexual orientation, against federal grantees that deny services to or otherwise discriminate against individuals and issued a new rule that seeks to eliminate those explicit protections.[19] In response, Lambda Legal and Democracy Forward filed a lawsuit against HHS in March 2020 on behalf of three organizations serving vulnerable communities, Family Equality, True Colors United, and SAGE.[20]

Then, on June 12, 2020, in the middle of Pride month, during the COVID-19 pandemic, and on the anniversary of the Pulse massacre, Trump's HHS announced that it was rolling back regulations protecting LGBTQ+ people that had been promulgated by HHS in 2016 under the Affordable Care Act, notwithstanding their need and effectiveness.[21] As a result, Lambda Legal, in conjunction with LGBTQ+ health care providers, community centers, and membership organizations, filed a lawsuit to stop this dangerous and unlawful attempt to carve out LGBTQ+ people from the protections against discrimination in health care.[22]

Case Study: Effective Partnerships with LGBTQ+ Community Centers and Health Care Providers Prove Helpful to Stopping Anti-LGBTQ+ Attacks

Perpetrators of discrimination have repeatedly misused religion in an attempt to legitimize their actions and shield themselves from legal action. This is no less true in the health care context, where health care providers are being empowered to clench their fists and deny life-saving treatment to marginalized communities under the guise of religion, even in cases of emergency. Patients are being turned away in their most desperate and vulnerable times of need.

There is no better example of this than our litigation against the Trump administration's so-called "conscience" Rule, which invited health care providers (and anyone whose responsibilities are even tangentially related to patient care) to deny medically necessary health care treatment to patients on the basis of health care providers' "religious or moral" objections to treating those patients.[23] We are fighting for the survival of patients and frontline health care providers who are crucial for LGBTQ+ people and other marginalized communities. The Rule was scheduled to go into effect November 2019, but we won![24] We prevented this chilling Rule from taking effect, at least for now while the case is on appeal.

The Rule would tie the hands of affirming health care providers, including hospitals and LGBT community centers, and prevents them from enforcing nondiscrimination requirements against staff members who deny treatment to patients, if the staff member has a religious or other moral objection to treating the person. The Rule specifically singles out gender affirming care and reproductive health care.

We represent providers of last resort. The Los Angeles LGBT Center and Whitman-Walker Health, for example, treat patients suffering from life-threatening emergencies who were denied emergency care elsewhere and who arrive at their facilities with more acute medical conditions resulting from delay of treatment because of prior discrimination.[25] Our clients meet crucial needs in our communities by providing affirming treatment without judgment to populations that have been refused care elsewhere, fear going elsewhere, or have lost trust in the health care system because of prior discrimination.

Noncompliance with the Rule would risk our clients losing all of their federal funding—Medicaid, Medicare, Ryan White, all of it. In other words, if the Rule had taken effect, these places of last resort would have had to shut their doors.

The regulation lacks an emergency exception. This means that it prevents health care providers from insisting that their staff stabilize a patient in an emergency until a substitute staff member who does not have a religious objection to treating the patient is identified and arrives. In fact, the Department of

Justice conceded in open court that under the Rule, an ambulance driver could leave a patient to die in the middle of Central Park rather than transport them to the emergency room if the driver religiously objects to assisting the patient. During the COVID-19 pandemic, this Rule would have empowered that same ambulance driver to leave a transgender patient to die rather than transport that patient to a hospital for life-saving emergency medical intervention.

This health crisis solidified the importance of ensuring that we fight discrimination in health care. The LGBTQ+ community is uniquely vulnerable to complications from COVID-19,[26] and our clients have reorganized their practices to respond to the needs of our community during this pandemic. Whitman-Walker Health, a plaintiff in the case, has transformed its practice to offer in-person respiratory clinics and COVID-19 testing. Another plaintiff, the Los Angeles LGBT Center, which serves seventeen thousand patients per year, remained open for medical services during the crisis.

Had this Rule taken effect, these health care providers and community centers on the front lines of saving lives each and every day would have been gone. Without these health care providers, there would be nowhere that the LGBTQ+ community would be guaranteed nondiscriminatory emergency treatment for COVID-19.

These LGBTQ+ affirming providers do more than treat individual patients. They are also critical to protecting public health—and were so even before the COVID-19 pandemic. We cannot afford for them to close their doors. This is why we fought against the countless discriminatory rules that the Trump administration released.

Closing Thoughts

The COVID-19 crisis clarified that we need to stand united to ensure that health care is available and provided to all people, devoid of discriminatory barriers to care. We need to protect our providers of last resort who are at the front lines fighting COVID-19, and we need to fight to enforce existing laws and regulations that require *all* health care providers to provide equal and affirming care to all patients regardless of their gender identity or sexual orientation.

ABOUT THE AUTHORS

Jamie Gliksberg was a senior attorney at Lambda Legal Defense and Education Fund, Inc., where her work focused on First Amendment issues, particularly defending against the use of religion to unlawfully legitimize discrimination against LGBTQ+ people and people living with HIV. Her cases involved advocating for equal access to health care and child welfare services. Jamie was at the forefront of developing strategies for combating attempts to elevate discriminatory conscience objections over the needs of patients, including LGBTQ+ patients who are refused medical care on the basis of providers' religious beliefs. Jamie is now a partner and co-head of the litigation practice group at Croke Fairchild Morgan & Beres.

Omar Gonzalez-Pagan is a senior attorney and the health care strategist at Lambda Legal. As health care strategist, Omar has been a leading voice in the proper interpretation of health care nondiscrimination laws. He has authored numerous amicus briefs urging courts to adopt the most protective standards possible, as he did in Ballenger v. Providence Hospital, and was counsel in Simonson v. Oswego County and Kadel v. Folwell, challenging discriminatory exclusions of coverage for transgender employees' transition-related health care. Omar is also lead counsel in Conforti v. St. Joseph's Healthcare, where he represents a transgender man denied a hysterectomy by a Catholic hospital.

NOTES

1   Holly Yan, Steve Almasy, and Jay Croft, "Coronavirus Has Killed More Than 100,000 People Across the US," CNN, May 27, 2020, accessed January 7, 2022, https://www.cnn.com/2020/05/27/health/us-coronavirus-wednesday/index.html; US Center Disease Control, "CDC Confirms Possible Instance of Community Spread of COVID-19 in U.S," February 26, 2020, accessed January 7, 2022, https://www.cdc.gov/media/releases/2020/s0226-Covid-19-spread.html; John Hopkins, "COVID-19 Dashboard by the Center for Systems Science and Engineering (CSSE)," accessed January 7, 2022, https://coronavirus.jhu.edu/map.html.

2   Kerith Conron and Shoshana Goldberg, "LGBT People in the US Not Protected by State Non-Discrimination Statutes," UCLA Williams Institute, April 2020, accessed January 7, 2022, https://williamsinstitute. law.ucla.edu/publications/lgbt-nondiscrimination-statutes; "The Lives & Livelihoods of Many in The LGBTQ Community Are at Risk Amidst COVID-9 Crisis," Human Rights Campaign Foundation, accessed January 7, 2022, https://tinyurl.com/ybo3zxx8.

3   *When Health Care Isn't Caring: Lambda Legal's Survey of Discrimination Against LGBT People and People with HIV* (New York: Lambda Legal, 2010), 5, accessed January 7, 2022, https://tinyurl.com/2p9cjfe9.

4   Shabab Ahmed Mirza and Caitlin Rooney, "Discrimination Prevents LGBTQ People from Accessing Health Care," Center for American Progress, January 18, 2018, accessed January 7, 2022, https://tinyurl.com/3ca92874.

5   S.E. James, J.L. Herman, S. Rankin, M. Keisling, L. Mottet, and M. Anafi, *The Report of the 2015 US Transgender Survey* (Washington, DC: National Center for Transgender Equality, 2016), accessed January 7, 2022, https:// transequality.org/sites/default/files/docs/usts/USTS-Full-Report-Dec17. pdf.

6   "The Lives & Livelihoods of Many in the LGBTQ Community Are at Risk Amidst COVID-19 Crisis," Human Rights Campaign Foundation, accessed January 17, 2021, https://tinyurl.com/yc25z4vs; *Ana Hernández (Equality Federation) and Oliver Stabbe (Lambda Legal)*, "The Deadly Cost of COVID-19 for LGBTQ+ Youth," June 4, 2020, accessed January 7, 2022, https://www.lambdalegal.org/blog/20200604_lgbtq-youth-covid-19; Lambda Legal, "The Cost of COVID-19 for LGBT Older Adults," April 28, 2020, accessed January 7, 2022, https://www.lambdalegal.org/blog/ lgbt-older-adults-seniors-elders-coronavirus.

7   American Progress and Movement Advancement Project and Movement Advancement Project, *Paying an Unfair Price: The Financial Penalty for Being Transgender in America* (Washington, DC: Center for American Progress and Movement Advancement Project, 2015), 5, accessed January 7, 20222, http://www.lgbtmap.org/file/paying-an-unfair-price-transgender. pdf.

8   Robert Steinbrook, "Contact Tracing, Testing, and Control of COVID-19—Learning from Taiwan," *JAMA Intern Med.* 180, no. 9, (September 2020), accessed January 7, 2022, https://jamanetwork.com/journals/ jamainternalmedicine/fullarticle/2765640.

9   "Equality Maps: Healthcare Laws and Policies," Movement Advancement Project, accessed January 7, 2022, https://www.lgbtmap.org/equality-maps/ healthcare_laws_and_policies.

10 "Equality Maps: State Nondiscrimination Laws," Movement Advancement Project, accessed January 7, 2022, https://www.lgbtmap.org/equality-maps/non_discrimination_laws.

11 42 U.S.C. § 18116.

12 81 FR 31375–Nondiscrimination in Health Programs and Activities, *Federal Register* 81, no. 96 (May 2016), accessed January 7, 2022, https://www.federalregister.gov/documents/2016/05/18/2016-11458/nondiscrimination-in-health-programs-and-activities; Bostock v. Clayton County, Georgia, no. 17–1618 (June 15, 2020).

13 Sharita Gruberg and Frank J. Bewkes, "The ACA's LGBTQ Nondiscrimination Regulations Prove Crucial," Center for American Progress, March 7, 2018, accessed January 7, 2022, https://tinyurl.com/2p97e5pn.

14 Complaint, Kadel v. Folwell, No. 1:19CV272, 2020 WL 1169271 (M.D.N.C. March 11, 2020) (No. 1); Flack v. Wisconsin Department of Health Services, 395 F. Supp. 3d 1001 (W.D. Wis. 2019); Boyden v. Conlin, 341 F. Supp. 3d 979 (W.D. Wis. 2018); Complaint, Simonson v. Oswego County, Case No. 5:17-CV-1309-MAD-DEP (N.D.N.Y., Stipulation filed August 23, 2017) (No. 1); "Victory! Lambda Legal Obtains Settlement for Oswego County Transgender Employee Denied Coverage for Transition-Related Care," Lambda Legal, accessed January 7, 2022, https://www.lambdalegal.org/news/ny_20180821_victory-settlement-for-oswego-county-transgender-employee.

15 Prescott v. Rady Children's Hosp.-San Diego, No. 16-CV-02408-BTM-JMA, 2018 WL 2193649 (S.D. Cal. May 11, 2018); Rumble v. Fairview Health Servs., No. 14-CV-2037 (SRN/FLN), 2016 WL 4515922 (D. Minn. August 29, 2016); *see also* Complaint, Conforti v. St. Joseph's Healthcare Sys., Inc., No. 217CV00050CCCCLW (D.N.J. January 22, 2020) (no. 1).

16 Protecting Statutory Conscience Rights in Health Care; Delegations of Authority, 84 FR 23170 (US Department of Health & Human Services 2019).

17 Complaint, County of Santa Clara v. Azar II, No. 3:19-cv-02405-WHA (N.D. Cal. 2019) (No. 1).

18 City & Cty. of San Francisco v. Azar, 411 F. Supp. 3d 1001 (N.D. Cal. 2019), appeal dismissed sub nom. City and County of San Francisco v. Azar II, et al., County of Santa Clara, No. 20-15398, 2020 WL 3053625 (9th Cir. June 1, 2020).

19 Notification of Nonenforcement of Health and Human Services Grants Regulation, 84 FR 63809 (US Department of Health & Human Services 2019).

20 Corrected Complaint, Family Equality v. Azar II, No. 1:20-cv-02403-MKV (S.D.N.Y. April 1, 2020) (No. 22).

21 "HHS Finalizes Rule on Section 1557 Protecting Civil Rights in Healthcare, Restoring the Rule of Law, and Relieving Americans of Billions in

Excessive Costs," HHS.gov, June 12, 2020, accessed January 7, 2022, https://www.hhs.gov/about/news/2020/06/12/hhs-finalizes-rule-section-1557-protecting-civil-rights-healthcare.html.

22   "UPDATE: Lambda Legal & HRC both announce plans to sue over ACA change," Dallas Voice, June 12, 2020, accessed January 7, 2022, https://dallasvoice.com/breaking-hrc-to-sue-trump-administration-over-discriminatory-aca-change; Complaint, Whitman-Walker Clinic, Inc. v. US Dep't of Health & Human Servs., No. CV 20-1630 (JEB) (D.D.C. filed June 22, 2020).

23   Litigation in collaboration with the Center for Reproductive Rights, Americans United for the Separation of Church and State, and pro bono counsel at Mayer Brown, and the County of Santa Clara. Lambda Legal, "County of Santa Clara v. HHS," accessed January 7, 2022, https://www.lambdalegal.org/in-court/cases/county-of-santa-clara-v-hhs.

24   City & County of San Francisco v. Azar, 411 F. Supp. 3d 1001, 1005 (N.D. Cal. 2019), appeal dismissed sub nom. City and County of San Francisco v. ALEX M. AZAR II, et al.; County of Santa Clara, et al., No. 20-15398, 2020 WL 3053625 (9th Cir. June 1, 2020).

25   Declaration of Naseema Shafi, County of Santa Clara v. Azar II, No. 5:19-cv-2916 (N.D.Cal. filed June 11, 2019), accessed January 7, 2022, https://tinyurl.com/ya3o8hmc; Declaration of Randy Pumphrey, County of Santa Clara v. Azar II, No. 5:19-cv-2916 (N.D.Cal. filed June 11, 2019), accessed January 7, 2022, https://preview.tinyurl.com/y8qqvzul; Declaration of Sarah Henn, County of Santa Clara v. Azar II, No. 5:19-cv-2916 (N.D.Cal. filed June 11, 2019), accessed January 7, 2022, https://tinyurl.com/y7ssnpsl; Declaration of Darrel Cummings, County of Santa Clara v. Azar II, No. 5:19-cv-2916 (N.D.Cal. filed June 11, 2019), accessed January 7, 2022, https://tinyurl.com/y7lwuj7c; Declaration of Robert Bolan, County of Santa Clara v. Azar II, No. 5:19-cv-2916 (N.D.Cal. filed June 11, 2019), accessed January 7, 2022, https://tinyurl.com/ycvk5o8s; Declaration of Ward Carpenter, County of Santa Clara v. Azar II, No. 5:19-cv-2916 (N.D.Cal. filed June 11, 2019), accessed January 7, 2022, https://tinyurl.com/ycoxoxjh.

26   Hernández and Stabbe, "The Deadly Cost of COVID-19 for LGBTQ+ Youth;" Lambda Legal, "The Cost of COVID-19 for LGBT Older Adults."

FROM GLORYHOLES TO VACCINE ADVOCACY: THE JOURNEY OF QUEER HEALTH ACTIVISM DURING COVID-19

Adrian Shanker

I'll never forget the day in June 2020 when the New York City Department of Health and Mental Hygiene (NYC DOH) published a guidance clarifying that gloryholes are safer than kissing.[1] This was just part of the journey of queer health activism during the COVID-19 pandemic.

Queer communities, like all communities, were thrust into uncertainty in March 2020 when it became clear that COVID-19 was a serious and dangerous virus, one that would certainly change our lives and our communities for the short term, with unknown long-term implications. When the whole world was thrust headfirst into chaos, it was difficult to ask for one minoritized and historically excluded community to be prioritized. Perhaps especially with limited or no data to demonstrate the disparities LGBTQ+ communities were facing. The journey of queer health activism during COVID-19 was one of searching for answers to questions we didn't know to ask yet. This was the evolution of activism through uncertain times.

After years of advocacy by queer community leaders, many hospitals and public health agencies were on the brink of updating their IT systems to include data fields that would finally, accurately count LGBTQ+ people in public health data. Then, all of a sudden, in the midst of a global pandemic, our queer communities learned that those IT upgrades hadn't been completed yet.

This was the story I heard again and again as I called hospitals and health agencies to plead with them to *please* collect demographic data on the LGBTQ+ community's experiences with COVID-19.[2]

Close to immediately at the start of the pandemic's first breach into the United States, the Centers for Disease Control and Prevention (CDC) mandated that state departments of health collect race and ethnicity demographic data related to COVID-19. But without a mandate for sexual orientation and gender identity data collection, the LGBTQ+ community would be left behind, with no data to prove what the CDC later confirmed to be true: LGBTQ+ people live with increased risk for the worst effects of COVID-19.

The sense of urgency was clear. When we aren't counted, it means we don't count. When there is no data, there is no way to demonstrate the community's needs. In moments of pandemic-related panic, the lack of data felt intentional, even though we all knew it wasn't.

Frequently, people would ask whether there were LGBTQ+ community disparities related to COVID-19. Of course, we had access to troves of data that demonstrated why LGBTQ+ communities were living with unique vulnerabilities to COVID-19, for example, higher smoking rates, higher incidence of cancer, and unsuppressed HIV, as well as barriers to health care and outright discrimination. But the truth was that we simply didn't have the data to know if there were disparities in COVID-19 infections, hospitalizations, or mortality.

When activists asked why these data weren't available, the weird and unfortunate response was "because of the IT systems."

I've been a queer community activist for years. I'm used to hearing government agencies and hospital networks say "no" to seemingly simple requests from the LGBTQ+ community, but even I was surprised that the issue wasn't due to a lack of political willpower, a lack of a desire to receive data on health disparities, or a lack of prioritization of health equity. It was simply "because of the IT systems."

As queer activists we have grown accustomed to learning just enough to be dangerous about many issues in order to be the strongest advocates we can be. ACT UP and Treatment Action Group activists learned more about pharmacology than many of them thought they would ever need to know in order to take on the government health bureaucracies and the pharmaceutical industry in the 1980s and 1990s and to demand that the government and the industry prioritize people living with HIV/AIDS. Many of us remember the last few years of the marriage equality fight when we were learning constitutional law on the internet because of the felt sense of urgency to tweet in real time and with authority about the seemingly daily victories in courts across the country. So it was, six weeks into the worst global health crisis in a century, that LGBTQ+ activists started to learn about IT systems, such as electronic health records and electronic public health reporting systems, just enough so we could talk to the hospitals and public health agencies to plead with them to add data fields to track LGBTQ+ COVID-related disparities.

Pennsylvania was the first. Dr. Rachel Levine, a transgender woman with a background in pediatrics, was Pennsylvania's secretary of health. Thrust into the daily spotlight at the start of the pandemic with frequent press conferences where she offered her daily reminders to help Pennsylvanians stay safe from COVID-19, Dr. Levine became a household name in Pennsylvania. Her daily press briefings exuded calm leadership and modeled data-informed decision-making at a time when more was unknown than was known about the rapidly spreading virus.

On April 13, 2020, twenty-six organizations led by the National LGBT Cancer Network and Bradbury-Sullivan LGBT Community Center wrote to Dr. Levine asking her to track sexual orientation and gender identity within Pennsylvania's

COVID-19 infection, hospitalization, and mortality data tracking systems. We wrote:

> [E]arly epidemiological analyses have spotlighted disparities in death rates for both African American and Latinx populations; these are exactly the type of analyses that also need to be conducted for the LGBT population. In order to do so, it is critical that hospitals and testing sites collect LGBT demographic data from COVID-19 patients (testing results, hospitalizations, and mortality). Without these data, efforts to limit exposure for the LGBT community through behavioral change (including community adherence to the sound direction from PA Department of Health and the CDC), as well as clinical efforts to improve care for adversely impacted populations, will be limited.

Naively, we thought it would be a quick fix. That a trans woman with authority to make the changes could do so quickly and uneventfully. But those damn IT systems frustrated the process of necessary and immediate change. We also learned that mortality data would need to be collected by independently elected county coroners, and in a purple state with sixty-seven counties (many of which are deep red counties less inclined to prioritize queer data collection) this would simply not be possible. But on May 13, 2020, exactly one month later, Pennsylvania governor Tom Wolf announced that the commonwealth would become the first in the country to collect sexual orientation and gender identity demographic data related to COVID-19 infections. It was a win!

But data collection efforts around sexual orientation and gender identity weren't complete with infection data. The next step was to ensure that the state's contact tracing process incorporated sexual orientation and gender identity demographic data collection fields as well. Luckily for advocates, the COVID-19 contact tracing process was in its infancy, and the state Department of Health was able to add these data fields into both the contact tracing app and the phone script contract tracers would utilize when reaching out to people to let them know they may have been in close contact with someone newly diagnosed with COVID-19. However, this addition required training for all of Pennsylvania's contact tracers to ensure that they would understand and feel comfortable asking questions about sexual orientation and gender identity. Between July 2020 and January 2021, Bradbury-Sullivan LGBT Community Center trained more than 1,200 contact tracers working for the Pennsylvania Department of Health, Philadelphia Department of Public Health, Erie County Department of Health, and Allentown Health Bureau. It was another win!

Inspired by the "Sex during COVID-19" guidance from NYC DOH, Pennsylvania activists rolled up our sleeves for the next level of queer health activism during COVID-19. On June 8, 2020, NYC DOH updated their March 2020 "Sex during COVID-19" guidance with new information to help stop the spread of COVID-19. The sex-positive document encouraged harm reduction strategies to prevent the spread of COVID-19. In one section, the document reads, "Make it a little kinky: Be creative with sexual positions and physical barriers, like walls, that allow sexual contact while preventing close face to face contact."[3] The guidance also encouraged harm reduction through limiting the number of partners and encouraged sex workers to take their business online through subscription-based fan platforms or "sexy zoom parties." This guidance was a model for the nation.

Pennsylvania is significantly more conservative than New York City, but buoyed by the enthusiasm of our recent data collection victory we knew what was possible. We also knew the political realities of our purple state and the challenge in navigating such policies. Among Pennsylvania's sixty-seven counties, there are fewer than a dozen municipal or county Health Bureaus. We knew that if a few of them adopted a sexual health guidance that the state Department of Health would follow. We started with the Erie County Department of Health. Erie is known as a blue dot in a sea of red, the one progressive city in otherwise conservative and rural northwest Pennsylvania. In former president Trump's failed reelection campaign, he even lamented needing to visit Erie to shore up support in western Pennsylvania (Biden ended up winning Erie County, and Pennsylvania, and, of course, the presidency.)

We started with Erie because of, not in spite of, the political realities. We wanted to demonstrate that sexual health during COVID-19 was not some liberal promotion of gloryholes, but, rather, that it was essential community health information that many people needed. The Erie County "Sex during COVID-19" guidance states:

> [S]ex is a normal part of life and should always be with the consent of all parties. This document offers strategies to reduce the risk of spreading COVID-19 during sex. Decisions about sex and sexuality need to be balanced with personal and public health. During this extended public health emergency, people will and should have sex. Consider using harm reduction strategies to reduce the risk to yourself, your partners, and our community.[4]

Shortly after Erie County, the City of Allentown Health Bureau followed with guidance of its own. Allentown's population is 43 percent Latinx, so the city Health Bureau translated their guidance into Spanish. Allegheny County's Health Department followed suit. Somewhere along the way Philadelphia's Department of Public Health released its guidance, followed by suburban Montgomery County. Finally, on October 7, 2020, the Pennsylvania Department of Health released statewide guidance, which said "All Pennsylvanians should stay home as much as possible and minimize contact with others to reduce the spread of COVID-19. During this extended public health emergency consider utilizing risk reduction strategies to protect your health and the health of your sex partner(s)."[5]

The win was not without controversy: Republican state senator Camera Bartolotta, who represents a rural community in Washington County, in southwest Pennsylvania, wrote on her Facebook page on December 15, 2020, "Here is your government telling you how to 'stay safe' from Covid during an orgy." Of course, Senator Bartolotta was wrong about the importance of sexual health information during a public health crisis, but some politicians can't be bothered with facts that get in the way of their rhetoric.

Once the first vaccines were given emergency use authorization in the United States, advocacy shifted to looking at who would be prioritized. Former president Trump neglected his responsibility to create a national vaccine distribution plan and left states to create their own plans. In Pennsylvania, queer activists were looking to ensure that people living with HIV would be prioritized. Early versions of Pennsylvania's vaccine distribution plan did not include people living with HIV on the list of people with underlying health conditions for vaccine priority. As advocates, we wanted to change that. Bradbury-Sullivan LGBT Community Center formed a coalition that included the AIDS Law Project of Pennsylvania, the SERO Project, Philadelphia FIGHT Community Health Centers, Philadelphia's William Way LGBT Community Center, and Harrisburg's LGBT Center of Central Pennsylvania. On December 14, 2020, the six organizations wrote a joint letter to then Pennsylvania secretary of health Dr. Rachel Levine that said:

> [P]eople living with HIV have concerns and questions related to their risk of serious illness from COVID-19. Based on the data available, people living with HIV, particularly people with low CD4 cell count, a high viral load, and people not on effective HIV treatment (antiretroviral therapy) are at increased risk for severe

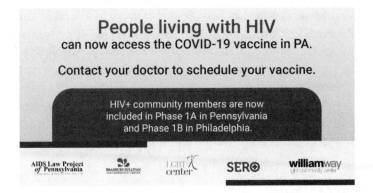

illness. We also know that people living with HIV are more vulnerable to respiratory infections when their HIV is not well managed. For these reasons it is very important to keep this population as safe as possible.

A coalition of Western Pennsylvania organizations led by the Hugh Lane Wellness Foundation echoed this call, as did the Human Rights Campaign in a December 21, 2020, letter to Governor Tom Wolf.

On January 19, 2021, Pennsylvania Department of Health announced a revised vaccine distribution plan and became the first state in the country to specifically identify people living with HIV as immediately eligible for the COVID-19 vaccine in Phase 1A of the state's vaccine distribution plan. It was another win!

Vaccine equity efforts didn't end there. The CDC had neglected to include sexual orientation and gender identity in their vaccine tracking system, and no states were doing it on their own. Of course, that meant that there would be no government data on vaccine hesitancy among LGBTQ+ people. Out Boulder, the LGBTQ+ community center in Boulder, Colorado, launched the first regional study to measure COVID-19 vaccine hesitancy within their local queer community. Bradbury-Sullivan LGBT Community Center and

Bryn Mawr College Graduate School of Social Work and Social Research followed suit with a statewide study in Pennsylvania. Kaiser Family Foundation released a national survey as well. But once again, the lack of demographic data tracking sexual orientation and gender identity on a government form meant that data would only be available if community organizations collected it themselves, and it would never be as complete a snapshot as if it was included on the government forms in the first place.

One thing that did become clear was the need for LGBTQ+ community vaccine clinics. Queer community centers across the country began offering them. This was complicated, as many LGBTQ+ centers are not set up to manage these types of health services, and the funding mechanisms that supported COVID-19 vaccine distribution in the US did not consider the cost for partnerships with community-based organizations. Yet during a period of four weeks, Bradbury-Sullivan LGBT Community Center arranged one thousand shots into arms at our vaccine clinics, and many other LGBTQ+ centers saw similar success. The Leonard-Litz LGBTQ+ Foundation privately funded vaccine clinics at five northeastern US LGBTQ+ community centers. Other organizations eventually received state or federal grants to distribute the vaccine. But many organizations were left to utilize their own limited resources to promote a lifesaving vaccine to our communities.

The journey of queer health advocacy throughout the first year of the COVID-19 pandemic was a constant challenge. When the needs are so great for the entire community, it is hard for policy makers, even those who support health equity, to prioritize it. Victories only happened because advocates fought for them. Queer songwriter Rena Branson wrote, "We will not underestimate our power any longer." This has to be the lesson activists take from COVID-19: in the words of Branson, "We know that together, we are strong."

ABOUT THE AUTHOR
Adrian Shanker's bio can be found on page 93.

NOTES

1   "Safer Sex and COVID-19," New York City Health, updated October 13, 2021, accessed January 7, 2022, https://www1.nyc.gov/assets/doh/downloads/pdf/imm/covid-sex-guidance.pdf.

2   Kevin C. Heslin and Jeffrey E. Hall, "Sexual Orientation Disparities in Risk Factors for Adverse COVID-19–Related Outcomes, by Race/Ethnicity—Behavioral Risk Factor Surveillance System, United States, 2017–2019," *Morbidity and Mortality Weekly Report* 70, no. 5 (February 5 2021):149–54, accessed January 13, 2022, https://www.cdc.gov/mmwr/volumes/70/wr/mm7005a1.htm.

3   "Safer Sex and COVID-19."

4   "Sex and Coronavirus Disease 2019 (COVID-19)," County of Erie Department of Health, accessed January 17, 2021, https://eriecountypa.gov/wp-content/uploads/2020/05/Sex-and-Coronavirus-Disease-2019.pdf.

5   "Safer Sex and COVID-19," Pennsylvania Department of Health, accessed January 17, 2022, https://www.health.pa.gov/topics/disease/coronavirus/Pages/Guidance/Sexual-Health.aspx.

≡

BUILDING OUR QUEER AND QUARANTINED SEXUAL WORLDS
Emmett Patterson

> I thought then
> Of holding you
> As a political act. I
> May as well have
> Held myself.
> —Jericho Brown, excerpt from "Stand"

> How would we organize and move our communities if
> we shifted to focus on what we long for and love, rather
> than what we are negatively reacting to?
> —adrienne maree brown, *Pleasure Activism*

Three months passed without grabbing my faithful bottle of poppers and trotting off to my hookup's house a few blocks away. Had I known it would be my last sexual foray into the outside world, maybe I would have taken more advantage of the moment. When discussing writing this chapter, my partner Rodrigo and I shared similar sentiments with each other. Our open relationship to unabashedly flirt, connect with, and fuck other people is an expression of our queerness. In a moment where we are both choosing to protect each other by forgoing sex outside of our household, I found myself mourning life where I felt at my most sexually liberated.

In the past few years, sexual liberation has become a framework through which I can view how the kind of sex I

want and have intertwines with my whiteness, my trans identity and queerness, my disabilities, my body size, and so many
more parts of me. A continuous process of growing and reflect-
ing, I have realized that sexual liberation is a road unpaved, one
that sharply turns as the potholes of shame and trauma litter
the path. Early on in understanding my transness, I maintained
social distancing before it was cool. Even though I had just
turned eighteen and headed off to a university in one of the
gayest cities in the US, I completely avoided gay sexual spaces,
fearing rejection and violence from cis men. I found myself
assessing risks and choosing celibacy to reduce potential harm.

Now, after finding myself strategically choosing celibacy
again, I am reassessing what safer sex and connection in lockdown might look like. As a sexual health activist, I feel that
we all have a stake in supporting each other and our desires
during a time of unprecedented uncertainty. For me, that
means: examining how queer people and our wisdom show
up in public health efforts during past and current pandemics;
understanding how abstinence-only messages miss the mark,
while pleasure-centered prevention could help; and ponder-
ing what opportunities we might have to mobilize our people
during the quarantine and after it is lifted.

Building a new reality in our quarantined roles leverages
our queer power garnered from past pandemics. Our queerness
is birthed from the vibrant lives of our queer ancestors, who
survived by connecting with each other through sex, radical
organizing, and collective care. This is not our first pandemic.
We queers have the tools, wisdom, and strength to envision these
new realities; meaning, we must remember how to curtail an
epidemic that thrives on our physical connection to each other
without sacrificing our real needs and desires for that connection.

Who Is the "Public" in Public Health?

Before I go straight into it (as if I can go *straight* into anything),
what do I mean by "public health," and how does sexual

liberation play a role? When stripping back public health to its essential components, we can see that it differs from a Western understanding of health care in two core ways: a focus on populations, rather than individuals, and prevention, instead of treatment. What I have all too quickly figured out while working in partnership with global activists is that public health frameworks alone are inadequate in describing and strategizing toward building a healthier world for queer people, often because we aren't seen as an integral part of the public itself.

Alexander McClelland, the cofounder of the Policing the Pandemic project, describes the way in which queer people and other marginalized people have been historically removed from public health:

> When we talk about public health, we have to think about who is the "public" in public health and whose health is being protected. And when we play that question out, we find that people living with HIV or queers are never the public in public health. They're always the subjects who the public is to be protected from. So we're framed as objects of risk that the public is to be protected from.[1]

To be marginalized is to be excluded from the very definition of public health and, thereby, its efforts. Black and Brown people, Indigenous peoples, queer people, trans people, disabled people, people living with HIV. . ., aren't we part of the public who needs protecting, too?

Recently, I have been questioning my place in the frame of "the public." If I were to map my identities, I would start with being a young, white, queer trans man. At the very beginning of the pandemic surge in the US, I was diagnosed with multiple autoimmune diseases and began biologic therapy to suppress my amped-up immune system. My disabled identity quickly became central in that map, because I instantaneously became both at-risk as an immunocompromised person but invisible in the pandemic as a young person. Every message coming from the US Centers for Disease Control and Prevention (CDC), the World Health Organization, and even Instagram was that young people need not worry; only older people and people with health conditions should be concerned. Even though official federal guidance did not mention people with chronic health conditions or disabilities, I felt the sting of ableism as I watched my peers flaunt their haircuts, crowds flock to the beach, and officials reopen their states despite COVID-19 infection and fatality rates continuing to grow.[2]

In thinking of public health, it's obvious that we cannot remove social conditions from our efforts. Public health leaders must not allow themselves to be comforted by "universalizing" approaches that don't take systemic violence into account. Even when it comes to intimacy and sex, the vast, specific needs that arise in historically marginalized communities remain central. In 2019, I co-led a group of trans and nonbinary community activists on a research project to outline steps toward sexual health and liberation for our communities. *A Blueprint for Trans and Non-Binary Sexual Health and Liberation* demonstrated that sexual health involves much more than STI testing and treatment; for trans and nonbinary participants, sexual health was "inextricable from overall mental and physical health," including commonly cited social determinants of health in public health discourse.[3] Racism, criminalization, ableism, xenophobia, economic and housing insecurity: these are significant aspects of our sexual health that often get essentialized out of public health. Public health leaders must not ignore the ways in which marginalization and sexual health interact over the course of this pandemic and how liberatory frameworks can describe and alter almost predetermined forces in our lives.

Throughout history, societies have focused on these social conditions by blaming the spread or origin of disease on marginalized people without acknowledging how systems of power remove access to lifesaving information to control one's health. For people impacted by the HIV and AIDS pandemic in the US, the 4H club named "homosexuals, Haitians, heroin users, and hemophiliacs" or rather "queer and trans people, Black people (and other people of color), people who use drugs, and people with disabilities" as both the most impacted in terms of infection and those responsible for the spread of HIV;[4] thus, these groups threatened the health of the privileged "public."

Societies continue to place marginalized people at odds with public health efforts in the name of protecting the "public." For example, in Seoul, South Korea, there was a threat to dox and out gay men and the LGBTQ+ community after a resurgence in new COVID-19 cases was linked to one man who visited LGBTQ+ bars and clubs.[5] At end of a three-month lockdown, as a way of curtailing the local epidemic, the UK effectively made hooking up illegal for partners who don't cohabitate, preventing queer people from having casual sex.[6] Race and ethnicity also play a vital role in scapegoating disease. There was a rise in anti-Asian discrimination and violence in the US,[7] with former president Trump's administration attempting to rename the disease "the Chinese virus,"[8] marking Asian Americans as targets and perpetuating racist violence from the top down. Finally, as the streets filled with protests demanding radical defunding of the police due to officers' murders of Black Americans, Black activists and their supporters braced for the blame of rising COVID-19 infections to fall on them, rather than on state officials who reopened too quickly before taking control of their local epidemics.[9]

#StayHome: Deconstructing the False Binary of Prevention versus Pleasure

At first, I bought into the simplicity of the abstinence-only approach when shelter in place began, both in terms of sexual and social interactions. I felt that if I had to stay home, everyone else would feel like they had an equal stake and would do so as well.

I was completely and utterly wrong. Like many others in the US, I have been conditioned to deprioritize my sexual desire and needs. My ideas began to shift after I read an essay by associate editor of *TheBody* Mathew Rodriguez that asked readers to think of intimacy and sex as an essential part of the human experience for many people, much in the way we considered essential services during the pandemic.[10] "Americans not only devalue sex; they put sex on a hierarchy—straight and procreative sex tops the pyramid, with a steep downward slope ending in the kind of sex being denied to many queer people now: sex for pleasure, including condomless anal sex."[11]

With the majority of people in the US having lived in some form of quarantine for almost a quarter of a year, we were long overdue to respond to the needs of queer people who desire touch, sex, and connection with each other and to plan for what comes next. The #StayHome push, an abstinence-only approach for our full lives, failed to take into account the aspects of queer connection that very much require us to leave our homes: whether we commune with our chosen family in breathy gossip or cruise our next regular in a cramped, musky bathhouse. Globally, queer people largely live with our blood families and cannot physically be with our community because of the threats of family rejection, criminalization, and violence. Rural queers in the US have far-reaching networks that extend beyond the confines of where we have been told to stay. Even for queer people who may themselves become strategically abstinent for a short time, lockdown orders without clear timelines and harm reduction strategies—such as those queer activists have crafted for STI prevention and drug use—do not address the balance of harms queer people must weigh: between exposure to a debilitating virus or the detriments of prolonged isolation.[12] When abstinence-only strategies like #StayHome are presented as the only viable option, queer people's physical, mental, and emotional health suffers.

At the bare minimum, this crisis makes clear that public health leaders need to acknowledge that self-isolation is unbelievably hard, that touch, desire, and sex can help alleviate the trauma stemming from internalized hatred, experiences of rejection, and acts of violence,[13] that sexual liberation for queer people means that we are free to define and realize our sexual experiences without stigma or outside intervention. Lockdown, abstinence-only messages and erasure of these concerns as not essential to public health are as great disservice to us as the pandemic drags on.

Public health leaders are beginning to take a stand. For example, in a recent op-ed, Dr. Julia Marcus, a professor of population medicine at Harvard Medical School, outlined the need to shift from the #StayHome message to a harm reduction focus, asserting that risk is a continuum, not a binary:

> Public-health experts have known for decades that an abstinence-only message doesn't work for sex. It doesn't work for substance use, either. Likewise, asking Americans to abstain from nearly all in-person social contact will not hold the coronavirus at bay—at least not forever.... #StayHome had its moment. The United States urgently needed to flatten the curve and buy time to scale up health-care capacity, testing, and contact tracing. But quarantine fatigue is real... [for] those who are experiencing the profound burden of extreme physical and social distancing.[14]

The biggest misconception of various voices in the quarantine conversation is that someone must stay at home or they will absolutely, 100 percent develop COVID-19. The pleasures of touch and prevention of a virus cannot be at odds moving forward. "If we ignore it, we are denying people's human needs," Dr. Marcus said in a follow-up interview. "If we say

'Stay home,' or 'You don't need sexual pleasure,' you're denying reality for people, and it's detrimental to our overall goals of public health."[15]

Queer Power Changes the Trajectory of an Epidemic—and the Rest of Our Lives

There is no silver lining to the insurmountable death, loss, displacement, and destabilization that COVID-19 wrought upon marginalized people globally. While most of us existed in some level of lockdown or decrease in our typical exposure to others, queer health organizations, activists turned social media influencers, social networks, and queer content creators found ways to address larger systemic issues, including and beyond COVID-19.

We must push public health institutions and leaders to react in real time to the wide swath of sexual health needs that queer people have with practical advice based in harm reduction. The New York City Department of Health and Mental Hygiene (NYC DOH) updated its already groundbreaking COVID-19 safer sex guidance to include information about consent, how long after a positive COVID-19 diagnosis it might be safer to have sex, and how to have safer group sex in lockdown.[16] Three months earlier, at the start of our quarantine, I could not have imagined typing these words and would have blamed it on the last hit of poppers: I see the opportunity for this pandemic to finally meet community needs for risk reduction guidance with the backing of health department and public health institutional legitimacy.

Why is NYC DOH's realistic stance so radical and unique in the world of public health? I believe it comes from the city's then deputy commissioner for the Division of Disease Control, Dr. Demetre Daskalakis, who penned the guidance. An HIV specialist and "an infectious disease expert as Tom of Finland would've imagined one—muscled, tattooed, leather-favoring," Dr. Daskalakis has "stood up to the mayor, convened webinars of sex workers, and issued guidance on everything from anilingus to proper testing protocols."[17] Tongue in cheek, he endorsed using jockstraps as no-sew face masks,[18] and the resulting tutorials prove our ingenuity.[19] Putting unapologetically queer people in charge of keeping people connected during this pandemic will allow us all to take control of our sexual health, using lessons that public health institutions have refused to learn in the past.

Other more decentralized technological institutions, such as social media and social networks, play a critical role in pandemic response for queer communities. Indigenous healers on Instagram and Twitter-certified health care professionals alike provided engaging ways for queer people to take control of our well-being. Well-known doctors in HIV circles have become social media influencers, with their approachable and accessible Facebook live Q&A sessions on meeting up with friends, family, and hookups.[20] Virtual spaces were claimed for queer pleasure, whether they were Zoom sex parties or virtual clubs, like Club Quarantine.[21] Centering pleasure in our quarantined worlds not only provides vital connection during a period of profound isolation but also opens access to that connection to parents of young children, people with disabilities, and older people for whom it is often inaccessible.

In addition, queer-specific dating app spaces like Grindr provided the richest soil for this critical act of connection to take place alongside of broader public health guidance. Throughout COVID-19 and other past epidemics,[22] our work at Grindr for Equality has leveraged the app's geolocation tools to connect users with HIV home tests in the US, queer mental health hotlines throughout Europe and North Africa, and updates on vital sexual health information that users were not receiving through their government ministries of health in local COVID-19 updates. There is certainly power in using technology to keep queer people connected to information and each other, but only in the hands of queer leaders who bring their life experiences into the action.

Queer activists and content creators took charge to disseminate vital information reminding quarantined queers of our ancestors' wisdom and strategies. Dr. Jaime Grant's *Just Sex* "emergency podcast" series highlighted stories from longtime activists to share kinky strategies on how to survive isolation.[23] JD Davids, founder of "The Cranky Queer Guide to Chronic Illness," wrote the first public guide on how to have sex during COVID-19 and hosted a roundtable of chronically ill and disabled "illders," healers, and medical providers to help chronically ill people prepare for COVID-19 long before health departments penned their guidances.[24] A collective of people with disabilities, fat people, old people, people with HIV/AIDS or other illnesses, and people of color launched #NoBodyIsDisposable, a campaign against discrimination in COVID-19 triage that leads to the premature death of individuals deemed not valuable in the ableist, racist, and ageist medical industrial complex.[25] Finally, an ongoing amfAR study and real-time data dashboard shows the devastating impact COVID-19 has on Black Americans—including gay, bi, queer, and same gender–loving men who already face the burden of lifetime HIV diagnoses—hoping that publicizing the COVID-19 race/ethnicity data that the CDC won't will lead to fund redistribution to protect Black communities during and post-COVID-19.[26]

We must continue to recognize that the many forms of violence we face in and out of the COVID-19 pandemic can be alleviated in weaving together our strategies. Put queer people in charge, and we can change the course of history.

All of us had a role to play in this pandemic. For queer people, deep in our bodies and minds lies the collective wisdom of ancestors longing for and loving each other with every radical step they took to stay connected through past pandemics. I feel this in my bones. It comforts me that we already know how to hold each other from afar, envision and enact new realities, and rise up to demand justice for our dead and dying. We are tasked to reach within ourselves and bring our desires out into the open and into our many roles in this moment. This pandemic, like those of our past, will require us to adapt and respond in real time. But isn't that what our queerness feels like? Fluidity, grace, and a desire to work toward a day when all will be well.

As the pandemic changed, so did we.

ABOUT THE AUTHOR

Emmett Patterson is a health activist, a writer, and the associate director of Building Healthy Online Communities. As the former global health projects manager of Grindr for Equality, he led the dating app's COVID-19 response, connecting the app's global user base with critical updates on the pandemic, safer sex information, and local support services. Over his career, he has worked in partnership with global activists in Latin America, Eastern Europe, the Middle East, North Africa, and North America on projects related to HIV home testing, migrant health, and trans and nonbinary sexual liberation. His writing on queer and trans health has recently been featured in *Out*, *The Advocate*, TheBody, and a book of essays, *Bodies and Barriers: Queer Activists on Health* (PM Press, 2020). He attributes his commitment to sexual health and liberation for himself and others to the wisdom of a lineage of HIV and AIDS, racial justice, and disability justice activists.

NOTES

1   Alexander McClelland, "Policing the Pandemic," *pinko*, May 13, 2020, accessed January 17, 2022, https://pinko.online/web/policing-the-pandemic.

2   Sarah Mervosh, Jasmine C. Lee, Lazaro Gamio, and Nadja Popovich, "See How All 50 States Are Reopening," *New York Times*, July 1, 2021, accessed January 17, 2022, https://www.nytimes.com/interactive/2020/us/states-reopen-map-coronavirus.html.

3   Anand Kalra, Emmett Patterson, Tori Cooper, Teo Drake, Shaan Lashun, and Kiara St. James, *A Blueprint for Trans and Non- Binary Sexual Health and Liberation* (Washington, DC: Grindr for Equality, 2020), accessed January 13, 2022, https://www.grindr.com/g4e/0422_G4E-TSH_Report-English.pdf.

4   Mathew Rodriguez, "COVID-19 and HIV Are Not the Same. But They're Similar in Many Ways That Matter," TheBody, April 9, 2020, accessed

January 13, 2022, https://www.thebody.com/article/covid-19-aids-not-same-but-similar-in-many-ways.

5   Michelle Kim, "Gay Men Outed in South Korea After COVID-19 Outbreak in LGBTQ+ Bars," them, May 11, 2020, accessed January 13, 2022, https://www.them.us/story/gay-men-outed-in-south-korea-after-covid-19-outbreak-in-lgbtq-bars.

6   Rachel Thompson, "Sex with Someone You Don't Live with Is Now Illegal in the UK," Mashable, June 2, 2020, accessed January 13, 2022, https://mashable.com/article/sex-ban-england-coronavirus.

7   N. Jamiyla Chisholm, "Asian Americans Report Hundreds of Racist Incidents in Less Than Two Weeks," Colorlines, March 27, 2020, accessed January 13, 2022, https://www.colorlines.com/articles/asian-americans-report-hundreds-racist-incidents-less-two-weeks.

8   Jérôme Viala-Gaudefroy and Dana Lindaman, "Donald Trump's 'Chinese Virus': The Politics of Naming," Conversation, April 21, 2020, accessed January 13, 2022, https://theconversation.com/donald-trumps-chinese-virus-the-politics-of-naming-136796.

9   Rob Davidson, Twitter post, June 5, 2020, 6:07 p.m., accessed January 13, 2022, https://twitter.com/drrobdavidson/status/1269028078304612353.

10   Mathew Rodriguez, "We Need a Plan for How to Have Casual Sex Again," TheBody, May 28, 2020, accessed January 13, 2022, https://www.thebody.com/article/casual-sex-covid-19.

11   Ibid.

12   "Lockdown Sex Ban Could 'Break the Chain' on HIV" (press release), Terrence Higgins Trust: Together We Can, June 4, 2020, accessed January 14, 2022, https://www.tht.org.uk/news/lockdown-sex-ban-could-break-chain-hiv; Roger Pebody, "A Quarter of Gay Men Report Casual Sex during UK Lockdown," aidsmap, June 11, 2020, accessed January 14, 2022, https://www.aidsmap.com/news/jun-2020/quarter-gay-men-report-casual-sex-during-uk-lockdown.

13   Felipe Flores, "Is Sex on Hold in the Queer Community during COVID-19?" San Francisco AIDS Foundation, May 4, 2020, accessed January 14, 2022, https://www.sfaf.org/collections/status/is-sex-on-hold-in-the-queer-community-during-covid-19.

14   Julia Marcus, "Quarantine Fatigue Is Real," *Atlantic*, May 11, 2020, accessed January 14, 2021, https://www.theatlantic.com/ideas/archive/2020/05/quarantine-fatigue-real-and-shaming-people-wont-help/611482.

15   Mathew Rodriguez, "We Need a Plan for How to Have Casual Sex Again," TheBody, May 28, 2020, accessed May 28, 2020, https://www.thebody.com/article/casual-sex-covid-19.

16   "Safer Sex and COVID-19" (press release), New York City Department of Health and Mental Hygiene, June 9, 2020, https://www1.nyc.gov/assets/doh/downloads/pdf/imm/covid-sex-guidance.pdf.

17   Matt Schneier, "The City's Tattooed Virus Expert Has Some Group-Sex Advice to Battle COVID-19," *Cut*, June 12, 2020, access January 14, 2022, https://www.thecut.com/2020/06/the-citys-tattooed-virus-expert-has-some-group-sex-advice.html.

18   Demetre Daskalakis, Twitter post, April 3, 2020, 12:22, p.m., unavailable January 14, 2022, https://twitter.com/drdemetre/status/1246110901478064129.

19   Emerson Collins, Twitter post, April 3, 2020, 6:44 p.m., accessed January 14, 2022, https://twitter.com/actuallyemerson/status/1246206902469459973.

20   Larry Buhl, "The COVID-19 Pandemic Is Turning More Doctors into Social Media Influencers," TheBodyPro, June 2, 2020, accessed January 14, 2022, https://www.thebodypro.com/article/covid-19-pandemic-turns-doctors-into-social-media-influencers.

21   Andrew Kahn, "Finding Life at Queer Virtual Sex Parties" (Outward podcast), March 24, 2020, accessed January 14, 2022, https://slate.com/human-interest/2020/03/sex-party-zoom-coronavirus-quarantine.html; "Inside Club Quarantine: The Future of Nightlife" (podcast), *Vice*, accessed January 14, 2022, https://www.youtube.com/watch?v=a-t-McubS0c.

22   "Inside Club Quarantine: The Future of Nightlife" (podcast), *Vice*, April 9, 2020, accessed January 14, 2022, https://www.youtube.com/watch?v=a-t-McubS0c.

23   Jaime M. Grant, "Emergency Podcast 1: Desire in the Time of the Coronavirus," *Just Sex: Mapping Your Desire*, March 24, 2020, accessed January 14, 2022, https://www.justsexpodcast.com/episodes/emergency-podcast-1-desire-in-the-time-of-the-coronavirus.

24   JD Davids, "How to Have Sex in the COVID-19 Coronavirus Pandemic," Cranky Queer, March 11, 2020, accessed January 14, 2022, https://thecrankyqueer.substack.com/p/how-to-have-sex-in-the-covid-19-coronavirus; "Coronavirus: Wisdom from a Social Justice Lens," *Healing Justice Podcast*, March 10, 2020, accessed January 14, 2022, https://irresistible.org/podcast/corona.

25   "Fight Discrimination in COVID-19 Triage," #NoBodyIsDisposable, 2020, accessed January 14, 2022, https://nobodyisdisposable.org.

26   Kenyon Farrow, "COVID-19 Is Devastating Black Communities. And amfAR Just Released New Data and a Website to Prove It," TheBodyPro, May 6, 2020, accessed January 14, 2022, https://www.thebodypro.com/article/covid-19-devastating-black-communities-amfar.

HOW LGBTQ+ CENTERS KEPT COMMUNITIES CONNECTED
Denise Spivak

Nobody was ready for a global pandemic, including LGBTQ+ community centers. But it happened. And they stepped up. Because when the going gets tough, LGBTQ+ centers keep on going!

First, some background. There are more than 250 LGBTQ+ centers across the US and Canada (even more around the globe). These centers are often the only staffed nonprofit LGBTQ+ presence in a community and the first point of contact for people seeking information, coming out, accessing services, or organizing for social change. Many LGBTQ+ centers provide some direct health services, including counseling, peer-led programs, support groups, and physical and mental health services, as well as diverse programming that reflects the communities they serve—communities that are racially and ethnically diverse, have concentrations of poverty, and include many transgender people. Serving more than 40,500 people every week, LGBTQ+ centers play a vital and multifaceted role in many communities across the country and around the world.

Many LGBTQ+ centers are brick-and-mortar operations, meaning they have physical space, they run in-person programs, offer in-person services, and provide drop-in space. Even many centers that operate without a space usually produce in-person events in rented or donated space, with the help of partner organizations. The bottom line is that LGBTQ+ centers are primarily face-to-face service providers, and one of the major impacts of the COVID-19 pandemic was that LGBTQ+ centers had to temporarily close their doors. Providing face-to-face services was just not an option.

The good news is that most LGBTQ+ centers were able to pivot and continue providing their face-to-face services—just not in person.

A few months before COVID-19 hit our communities in the United States, most LGBTQ+ centers could not have told you the difference between Zoom and Skype—or possibly what either of those even were! Even though as early as 2018 nearly three in ten LGBTQ+ centers offered some sort of online services, including live streaming of events, online social spaces for youth, and online chat programs, most of these organizations were not what one would call "tech-savvy" when it came to online programming.

In the span of a week, many of LGBTQ+ centers did extreme turnarounds. They altered their in-person service model and created virtual operations, taking their programs online, learning how to use Zoom, Facebook Live, Discord, QChat Space, and other streaming services.

Some moved quickly, but for others it took a little time. One LGBTQ+ youth center told me that the reason they were able to pivot so quickly and move their support programs to Discord within a week was because they had brought on a teen employee a short time before, and that person was able to give them a tutorial and help them. Had they not hired a teen onto their staff, they estimate it would have taken them a few more weeks to get up and running! However long it took, LGBTQ+ centers continued to connect the members of their community with information, with resources, and with each other.

As COVID-19 set in, LGBTQ+ centers noted current or expected increases in types of needs of clients or communities, demand for services or support from clients and communities, demand for existing and new programs, disruption of services for clients or communities, unplanned staff and volunteer absences, disruption of supplies or services from partners, and increased operational costs. More than 50 percent of LGBTQ+ centers reported that within a month or so of COVID-19 impacting their community they were providing services that directly supported the health or basic needs of those affected by the COVID-19 pandemic. Forty-five percent changed their operations or services so that they could more directly provide support to those involved in the COVID-19 response, and 20 percent reported providing a service that mitigates the spread of COVID-19. Larger LGBTQ+ centers, particularly those that offer medical services, remained open with modified operations. A number of LGBTQ+ centers also reported dedicating time to advocating for the health of their constituents, to make sure that they were able to access health care, stepping in when health care was challenged or denied and fighting discrimination head-on to ensure that LGBTQ+ people in their communities received much-needed care.

The other side of the coin was literally a lack of coins. While LGBTQ+ centers were finding new ways to support their community members, they were also trying to figure out how they were going to raise the money necessary to continue operating. The fundraising events that had come to provide such large chunks of funding for centers were in danger of being cancelled, as were Pride month events, fee-for-service programs, annual galas, and special fundraisers. By May 2020, these fears were realized, and events were cancelled, leaving most LGBTQ+ centers wondering how they were going to make up lost funds. Some organizations turned to online events, learning how to take their fundraisers and pride celebrations virtual. Others opted to postpone, hoping that things would improve, and events could be held at a later date.

While a good number of LGBTQ+ centers received federal assistance through the CARES Act, enabling them to bring back or retain employees and pay some bills, the long-term financial impact of COVID-19 on LGBTQ+ centers seemed uncertain.

For some, it meant business *not* as usual: adjusting and adapting as COVID-19 measures allowed, finding new sources of funding, and relying on consistent donors, supporters, and grantors. For others, it meant the end of business altogether.

LGBTQ+ community centers are the heart and soul of their communities—leading celebrations in good times, providing comfort in bad times, and providing services through the best and worst of times. Like the communities they serve, LGBTQ+ centers are resilient; they are the heart and soul of the LGBTQ+ movement and are vital to our current well-being and our dreams for the future. Whether they provide direct services, educate the public, or organize for social change, community centers work more closely with their LGBTQ+ constituencies and engage more community leaders and decision makers than any other LGBTQ+ network in the country.

So, what's next? Larger organizations, groups, and social influencers rallied to support centers during the pandemic through fundraisers and awareness, but for many centers the future is still uncertain. No doubt, when the "new normal" is realized, LGBTQ+ centers will not be the same. They will have experienced loss at some level, whether loss of family, friends, staff, constituents, and/or community members, and they will be forced to operate in a new way, impacted by health considerations, technological advancement, and financial changes. Nevertheless, LGBTQ+ centers will persist; they will go on as they have for over fifty years: serving, protecting, and celebrating our communities as only they can. The lesson of COVID-19 is that LGBTQ+ centers always show up to support the communities they serve.

ABOUT THE AUTHOR
Denise Spivak is the CEO of CenterLink: the association of LGBTQ+ community centers, where she has spent the past nine years working with center leaders. Denise joined CenterLink after working in the private sector for over twenty years in both broadcasting and management. She is a graduate

of Gettysburg College where she received her BA in psychology and holds a certification from BoardSource for nonprofit governance training. Denise was born and raised in the Washington, DC, area. After living in the mid-Atlantic for thirty years, she and her wife moved to Florida, where they currently reside.

CORONAVIRUS IS A DRAG: LGBTQ+ RESILIENCE AND LEADERSHIP THROUGH DRAG ARTS

Sigfried Aragona

Drag artists—queens, kings, monsters, genderbenders—are impressively resourceful, creative, and resilient people. As drag artists, we are familiar with looking into the face of trauma, grief, anxiety, and hardship. Naturally, in response, we paint a whole new face on negativity. Ironically, in the art of impersonation and transformation, we find our most authentic and empowered sense of self, fueled by an intrinsic motivation, as if our identities depended on it. Through this eclectic artform, drag performers embody their fantastical and ideal selves to move, entertain, and uplift their audiences. Drag shows provide a carefree and campy ambiance that is separate from the reality that exists in the outside world.

The start of the COVID-19 outbreak shook up our livelihoods. Everyone in the country was asked to contribute their cooperation, talents, and kindness. Health care professionals and other frontline workers continued to work tirelessly to care for the physical needs and health of their communities. As we all moved into our quarantine quarters, we faced new challenges that extended past boredom, and we sought ways to combat isolation, anxiety, and depression. As we battled the public health, mental health, and economic struggles that the rest of the country felt, our innovation as drag artists had to adapt as well.

Bars and restaurants closed, gigs were cancelled, resources were limited, and we were all asked to stay home. Full-time drag performers became unemployed with no certainty about the future of their drag careers. Some of my friends had to hide their drag while quarantined in the homes of unaccepting families. In the midst of the adversity, we whipped out our sewing machines, turned on our webcams, and exercised our creativity to new limits. We quickly accepted the reality of living in a pandemic and found our role as drag artists and performers to be the light during another difficult and fearful time.

The life of a queer person is fraught with experiences of loneliness, disappointment, anxiety, and suppression as a result of society's misconception and stigmatization of our gender identity and/or sexual orientation.[1] Queer artists are not foreign to inventing creative solutions to new challenges, setbacks, or opposition. In producing our art, drag artists reflect a form of queer leadership. We display utmost confidence in our appearance, behavior, and performance. We present our flamboyant and larger-than-life queer selves with no apologies. Our sheer presence is enough to make a statement, inspire someone, or provoke a dialogue—and we are armored in our wigs, makeup, and costumes to respond to the blunt end of any homophobia, transphobia, and ignorance aimed at our community.

The COVID-19 pandemic set our queer leadership skills and talents into motion. Mister Treats lives as a full-time drag performer/producer, costume designer, and teacher in Harrisburg, Pennsylvania. They shared that they couldn't "stand being idle, and really want[ed] to help the community" however they could.[2] With a generous heart and creative mind, Mister Treats demonstrated this queer leadership at the local level by donating more than one hundred masks to essential workers and immunocompromised individuals in their community.[3] Sushi, an iconic drag performer from Key West's "shoe drop," organized her drag troupe, 801 Girls, to donate more than 2,500 face masks to essential workers across the globe.[4] While not on the frontlines, the drag community

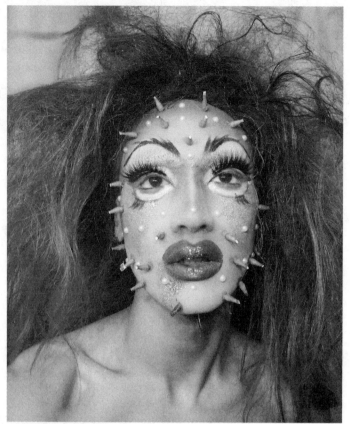

Drag artist Mandy Mango presenting as the coronavirus.

demonstrated that our craftmanship is not just worth glitz and glamour but has practical value that can protect and support other heroes in our community.

Our queer leadership and drag artistic skill set also extended into a different space. Queer artists and leaders, who were restricted from the physical LGBTQ+ spaces that they had carved out, generated virtual LGBTQ+ spaces during this time of isolation. Queer artists all over the country and across various levels of experience continued to produce their art despite the lack of income, in order to support their audiences through the uncertainty and fright. Nationally renowned drag artist and winner of the series *Dragula*, season 2 Biqtch Puddiń adapted the stage to a virtual drag show with suggested donations and tipping. Featuring drag artists across the globe, this digital adaptation entertained an audience of more than eight thousand people.[5]

Nina West continued her Drag Story Hour event online for children and families quarantined at home.[6] Local artists, such as Mister Treats and Glitter Douglas from Salisbury, Maryland, mobilized their local networks and resources to produce livestream drag shows during a time of required social distancing.[7]

Yet despite the shift in performance space and energy, our drag art continued in its spirit to entertain and move audiences. Glitter Douglas explained, "It was a more spur of the moment response. I can't stand being stagnant in performance. The [COVID-19 pandemic] has put new restrictions on what it means to perform. . . . It doesn't matter. Just keep moving forward."[8] Our almost instinctive reaction to our community crisis was to dive into our art, whether it was to foster our own well-being or the well-being of others. Drag art still provided a distracting and energizing opportunity to explore gender identity and self-expression. Drag artists, in our empowered selves, manifested our art with even more intention behind the concepts of our content. We aimed to entertain and relieve feelings of isolation by making people laugh. We did not just distract from the pandemic but led audiences in laughing *at* the pandemic. Flipping the script of the outbreak and its following events, COVID-19-themed content sought to hold a torch of optimism and humor to audiences and spectators. The category was COVID-19 Pandemic Palooza, and we stomped the runway with social media trends and challenges, punny song lyrics and mixes, and clever concepts for makeup and costumes. Our audiences were more *gagged* than the patients that had to be intubated. We provided comedy during the tragedy, understanding wholeheartedly the gravity of the pandemic

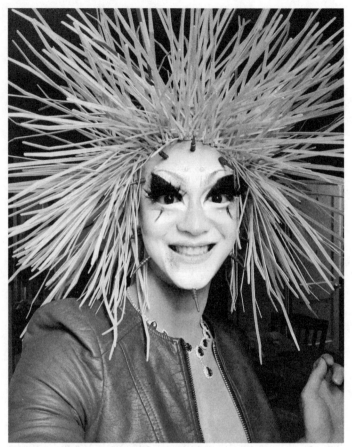

Drag artist Mandy Mango presenting as the coronavirus.

surrounding us. We were simultaneously improving our drag skill set and creating opportunities for laughter while in the mess of it all. "Drag performers carry so much magic and so much power. Whether it's deserved or not, a lot of people in the queer community look to us for inspiration, or even guidance," Mister Treats points out. They go on to say, "I feel more responsibility now than ever to continue being a positive inspiration for our community and to use that power to facilitate space for all of us in this new landscape."[9]

As with every profession during the COVID-19 outbreak, drag professionals had to adapt to the ongoing changes occurring every day. Our responsibilities as artists, entertainers, and queer leaders did not stop but multiplied in the face of this dilemma. Our history and experiences as LGBTQ+ people has thickened our skin and equipped us with our talents, resourcefulness, and intrinsic drive to uplift our communities. We demonstrated the artist's role in caring for the mental and emotional health of those in isolation and those working on the frontlines. Drag artists, specifically, modified our performance styles for videos and livestreams, juxtaposing the grim tone of news outlets and the media. We took comedic angles on hand hygiene, social distancing, working remotely, and the shortage of toilet paper. Some of us utilized our queer leadership to remind and educate people that consuming disinfectants is harmful and not preventative of infection, even if it was the advice of national presidential leadership. Our queer leadership was born from an adaptive mindset to persevere when the current systems in place cannot or will not serve us, when our communities have no place for us or when our families do not accept us. We build our own communities, find our loving families, and foster new traditions. Through these experiences, we forge the armor and paint (or makeup) the *mug* to confront the world and all its prejudices. Through all society's attempts to ignore LGBTQ+ existence, we survive and thrive by molding spaces that will validate us, our art, and our community—especially through a pandemic.

Our ability and motivation to sustain our art reflects this extraordinary grit that belongs to a community often viewed as fairies, freaks, and fags. While the feelings of seclusion and "lockdown" are all too familiar to the LGBTQ+ community, we showcase to the world and prove to ourselves that our negative experiences have not set us back but have pushed us to find our truest, strongest, most beautiful selves. This message is the sentiment embedded in every look, performance, and joke and stitched into every single mask sewn. In the 1980s and 1990s, drag artists ignited a light of resilience, hope, and community during the United States' public health battle against HIV/ AIDS.[10] While the LGBTQ+ community carries a heavy trauma from that history, we emerged knowing how to spring into action and strategize our strengths when crisis strikes. In the age of COVID-19, drag artists sprang into action once again to cast a broader light during the public health battle against COVID-19. When America looks back on this wild point in history, the nation will have to recognize that while the drag community knows how to throw shade, we are also a light in the dark.

ABOUT THE AUTHOR

Sigfried Aragona, RN, BSN, ACRN works as an ambulatory nurse in infectious diseases. Sigfried has been serving the HIV community in both rural and urban settings in various roles, including clinical case manager, sexual health nurse, and community educator. Sigfried also seeks to combat stigma and shame associated with sexual health and HIV through community education, drag programs, performances, and social media content as his drag queen persona, Mandy Mango (she/her). Sigfried utilizes this nurse-drag queen platform to increase awareness around LGBTQ+ health disparities and promote community wellness. Sigfried currently lives in Philadelphia, Pennsylvania, with his three cats: Sriracha, Wasabi, and Soy.

NOTES

1   Michael Hobbes, "Together Alone: The Epidemic of Gay Loneliness" Huffington Post, March 2, 2017, accessed January 14, 2022, https://highline. huffingtonpost.com/articles/en/gay-loneliness; Shainna Ali and Sejal Barden, "Considering the Cycle of Coming Out: Sexual Minority Identity Development," *Professional Counselor* 5, no. 4 (December 2015): 501–15, accessed January 14, 2022, https://tinyurl.com/3sycdnp6; Mayo Clinic Staff, "Health Concerns for Transgender People," Mayo Clinic, accessed January 14, 2022, https://www.mayoclinic.org/healthy-lifestyle/adult-health/ in-depth/transgender-health/art-20154721; "Lesbian, Gay, Bisexual, and Transgender Health," Office of Disease Prevention and Health Promotion, accessed January 14, 2022, https://www.healthypeople.gov/2020/ topics-objectives/topic/lesbian-gay-bisexual-and-transgender-health.
2   Hanniel Sindelar (aka Mister Treats), email interview, April 19, 2020.

3   Ibid.

4   Patrick Kelleher, "Meet the Drag Queens Taking on the Ultimate Sewing Challenge—Making Protective Equipment for Healthcare Workers," PinkNews, April 10, 2020, accessed January 14, 2022, https://tinyurl.com/2p9yhbsd.

5   Brittany Spanos, "As Gay Bars Close, Drag Shows Go Online," *Rolling Stone*, March 24, 2020, accessed January 14, 2022, https://www.rollingstone.com/culture/culture-features/virtual-drag-shows-coronavirus-pandemic-970347; Jael Goldfine, "Livestream This: A Digital Drag Show Hosted by Biqtch Puddin," *Paper Magazine*, March 16, 2020.

6   Bil Browning, "Coronavirus Can't Stop Drag Queen Story Time. It's Going Virtual Now," LGBTQ Nation, March 20, 2020, accessed January 14, 2022, https://www.lgbtqnation.com/2020/03/coronavirus-cant-stop-drag-queen-story-time-going-virtual-now.

7   Sindelar, email interview; Jacob Brittingham (aka Glitter Douglas), email interview, April 16, 2020.

8   Ibid.

9   Sindelar, email interview.

10 Vincent Chabany-Douarre, "From Fanny and Stella to Ru Paul's Drag Race: A Short History of Drag," History Extra, Immediate Media Company Limited, November 8, 2019.

≡

BREATHING IN SOLIDARITY
Zephyr Williams

Let's all pause and take a collective breath.
Inhale for 4...3...2...1.
Hold for 7...6...5...4...3...2...1.
and
Exhale for 8...7...6...5...4...3...2...1....

The first year of the COVID-19 pandemic was intense, a veritable game of social justice whack-a-mole. It felt like every time we started getting an ounce of control over one situation another one would pop up, laughing maniacally as we pivoted to restrategize. COVID-19 would have been enough of a challenge as we navigated the new normal of quarantine, social distancing, and Zoom meeting after Zoom meeting. Then came George Floyd, Breonna Taylor, Dion Johnson, and Tony McDade. All Black people. All murdered by cops. Enough was finally enough. Communities across the country rose up to face down the dynamics of power, privilege, and race and demanded a new way of life. The resounding message was clear. The tools of oppression are too costly to ignore or sustain any longer.

COVID-19 made visible what those of us on the ground, community organizations and activists alike, have known for years. Prisons and jails are dangerously overcrowded, unhygienic, violent, and dehumanizing institutions. It wasn't a question of if COVID-19 would spread through correctional facilities but when. Jails and prisons are not designed for people, let alone for preventing the spread of a deadly virus. Social distancing is near physically impossible in an eight by six–foot cell crowded with people. Meals are mostly communal, with incarcerated people seated elbow to elbow. Personal protective equipment and cleaning supplies were also in short supply. Frequent handwashing is difficult when soap is not readily available. Most people on the inside are not provided with soap; they must buy it from the commissary. During COVID-19, correctional facilities simply didn't have it. In many facilities, alcohol-based hand sanitizer is considered contraband.

Beyond that, incarcerated people, especially in local jails, cycle in and out; and correctional staff leave and return daily, often without screening. Testing was in short supply so it was hard to know exactly who did and did not have COVID-19. When incarcerated people were tested and found to be positive, they were often sent to solitary confinement. In general, there was a lack of basic protection and conflicting information, not only about COVID-19 but also about how it was spread. Incarcerated people were left to die. This is especially alarming given that people in these facilities are more likely to be immunocompromised due to age, HIV/AIDS, or other chronic health issues.

The COVID-19 pandemic was a wake-up call about these conditions inside correctional facilities for many people, one which also drove us to reassess how we serve our communities. Our understanding of the work remains unchanged, but how we plan to achieve our vision of liberation has changed. We were forced to reorient and strategize, map out our resources and needs, and form new collectives.

Like many other community organizations, Black & Pink rallied behind our people. We raised rapid response funds and resources through crowdfunding, mutual aid networks, and emergency grants. This allowed us to put money on our incarcerated people's books so they could purchase needed items.

We created networks of people inside, so that we could reach even more people. Bailing people out became a catch-22. If we got people out, where would they go? Couch surfing didn't seem like a viable option given the stay-at-home orders and the call for social distancing. How would they get groceries or find employment? We were caught between getting our people free and providing them stable and affirming access to the care and community that is needed upon release from incarceration.

We banded together with other organizations to demand a reduction in dangerous overcrowding by releasing the elderly, those with HIV/AIDS, other immunocompromised people, individuals with less than eighteen months left on their sentence, and pretrial detainees. The risk of carefully releasing people was vastly outweighed by the risk of leaving everyone inside. We demanded that jails and prisons prioritize the health and safety of incarcerated individuals by providing them with free hygiene and cleaning products, allowing for more phone calls, as visitations were shut down, and providing free testing, screening, and treatment of COVID-19. Given that the majority of COVID-19 clusters were inside correctional facilities, it was only a matter of time before those of us on the outside were impacted as well. Protecting people considered the least among us would ultimately protect all of us.

Post-COVID-19, will be a rare moment of opportunity. The mere fact that correctional facilities across the country were releasing incarcerated people in droves signaled that perhaps just reforming prisons isn't the answer. Maybe we shouldn't be incarcerating this many people in the first place. Perhaps the time has come to listen to the wisdom of prison abolitionists like Mariame Kaba, Angela Davis, Patrisse Cullors, and Ruthie Wilson Gilmore.

It's a much larger conversation to figure out just how millions of people got incarcerated in the first place and whether the prison system should be our answer. It's about more than just decarcerating as many people as possible to stave off a deadly virus. People are not only sentenced to time. They are sentenced to a lifetime of stigma, rejection from job opportunity after job opportunity, unstable housing, and roadblocks to necessities. Most will end up impoverished and without connection to care or affirming support upon returning home. This is state-sanctioned violence, discrimination, and neglect, a death sentence far outpacing the effects of COVID-19. Many of these people will come home. They are still our friends, our neighbors, and part of our community. They deserve better. We're all in this together.

We must act to take advantage of what might not have been possible prior to COVID-19. We know that there is no going back to normal or business as usual. Racism, homophobia, transphobia, misogyny, ageism, ableism, and other forms of oppression work together to keep people locked down and pushed out. Prison systems became our default, with a mentality of "by any means necessary." It translated into a callous disregard for human life during a crisis. We must ask ourselves: Was our way of bringing people to "justice" always this way? Can we move beyond reforms to something more restorative, more transformative?

We can, and we are. For those of us organizing in prison abolition spaces, it comes down to how we relate to one another as a people and a community. The way our prison system relates to people now is through retribution. Harm occurs, but the people involved in it are not centered in the process. People cause harm and people experience harm, but the state steps in to remedy it. Those who experience harm are not valued or heard, nor are those who cause it allowed to be accountable in a way that makes sense for the people who experience it. Acting through retribution doesn't allow for accountability or healing. The experience of harm is nuanced and complicated, because people are complex. Retribution is too simplistic a response to the breakdown in relationships that results from harm. Restoring these relationships through community support, active conversations, and inclusion offers a better solution.

COVID-19 offered a glimpse into this possibility. Even in the midst of the uncertainty and fear of a global pandemic, communities rallied around mutual aid practices, people sent one another care packages, handed out free weed, practiced physical social distancing with Zoom calls, and offered free self-care guidance like yoga practices and meditation, among other things. Unapologetic acts of love and service were happening before our governments stepped up.

Values of mutual aid and community care that organizations like ours and others have been advocating for and practicing took root in the everyday practices of communities. People figured out what safety looks like for themselves and determined their needs and how to meet them. Others in their community responded to these needs. People, whether they knew it or not, practiced transformative justice. A justice practice that is a Native way of life, and that, most recently, women of color, Black women in particular, drafted as an intentional blueprint to follow, was transforming communities across the country.

It became obvious that pain and violence are viruses themselves. Not only do they spread without corrective action, but, pointedly, punishment replicates the pain and violence. We have space for healing and meeting people where they are at home in our communities. We see them every day. Maybe we give a smile or a nod. Put people in cages, isolated and separated from communities, and we lose their humanity. We forget they too are worthy of respect and love. They too have inherent value. We must do better, folks—be better.

Transformative justice is about existing in a world centered on equity and access for all. It's about taking stock of our current institutions and ways of relating to each other and recognizing the "isms" (racism, ableism, classism, sexism, etc.) and "ics" (misogynistic, transphobic, homophobic, etc.) are really just a hoarding of power and privilege. Transformative justice is about change and healing. It's about having the courage to say: "I'm beautiful enough. Here are my resources, and here are my needs." Transformative justice asks of us some tough questions, but they are questions that are already being interrogated. How can we exist together recognizing we are all complicated beings? How do we unpack conflict and harm? How do we shift ideas of power so everyone can have the things they need to empower themselves?

We keep trying. We keep failing. We keep figuring it out. Achieving liberation through transformative justice is a marathon, not a sprint.

ABOUT THE AUTHOR

Zephyr Williams (any/no pronouns) is the deputy director for Black & Pink. Their experiences with the system as a gender-liberated person have propelled him toward community building, addressing marginalization, and challenging our ideas of justice. Zephyr works to dismantle the oppressive systems that perpetuate violence on the trans and queer community through a transformative justice practice. Through this lens, we can reignite that spark of courage within each of us that fans our flames of embodied worthiness and love. None of us are free until all of us are free. In xyr spare time, Zephyr can be found curled up with a good book, analyzing natal charts, having a dance break, or traveling the trails.

PROTEST AMID THE PANDEMIC
Michelle Veras

During the summer of 2019, just months before the first reported cases of COVID-19 in the United States, a group of Providence, Rhode Island, activists planned and carried out our city's first Dyke & Trans March for People of Color—we called ourselves and the event DTPOC PVD.[1] We aimed to create a space that would serve both as a celebration of our intersectional identities and a locus of resistance to the city's traditional Pride celebrations, which almost exclusively center the identities of white, cisgender, gay men. The event was a success, bringing together about a hundred people—and as I looked around I knew that I was among a group that could be a part of ushering in a new world.

As 2019 progressed, the feelings of community and solidarity I had experienced at the march in June began to fade. Rhode Island winters can be brutally cold and isolating. Living in a place where the sun sets before 4:30 in the afternoon often means spending six months of the year fighting off the physical and emotional impact of the dark and cold that feel all-encompassing. As with many in our queer family, the holidays can also take an emotional toll on me, and the final weeks of December brought the painful end of a relationship that had long sustained me. Couple that with images of Black and Brown folks murdered at the hands of police and what felt like new levels of racial, economic, and social injustices, and you could sense the collective desire to rid ourselves of all that 2019 had been.

I could not have imagined what 2020 would bring. Early in the year, I lost a dear friend, tragically and unexpectedly. He was only fifty, and losing him hit me hard. With his death I also lost a part of myself, a part of myself that I often felt only he could see. There are stories that so clearly illustrate the impacts of systemic racism, of health and economic disparities. For me, these moments often come when I see the effects play out in the lives of people in our community, as was the case with Roberto. I did not have a chance to pause and mourn his loss for long before the first cases of COVID-19 were reported in Rhode Island. In somewhat of a trance, I moved from my well-established routine—working in an office, going to the gym, sending a child to school every day, visiting friends—to what felt like a state of complete disconnection with no end in sight.

For me, not unlike others, the early weeks of the pandemic were permeated with uncertainty. The uncertainty seemed to extend from the more serious to the mundane. Would I lose my job? Would my son be okay? Would my brother, who is disabled and chronically ill, come down with the virus? Would my son return to school in the fall? What would the coming months look like? What would happen to Pride celebrations? What would happen to the 2020 DTPOC march?

Against the backdrop of the raging COVID-19 crisis, the state-sanctioned violence inflicted on Black and Brown communities did not let up. With each passing week, the list of Black men and BIPOC trans people lost to violence grew longer and longer. As organizers of the DTPOC march, we issued a statement on the murders and, out of an abundance of caution, canceled the 2020 march.

Weeks later, we reversed course and moved forward with plans to gather for a silent march, with a specific intention of remembering the Black trans lives we had lost to violence over the last year. With each passing day, the act of compiling an up-to-date list of their names felt unrelenting. We would finish the list on any given evening leading up to the event, only to wake up to news of another lost life to add to the list. Finally, on June 19, 2020, we gathered in the same location as we had the previous year. This time, we wore masks, encouraged physical distancing, and had plenty of hand sanitizer and extra masks on hand; COVID-19 safety measures had been the reason for our initial decision to cancel the gathering. In the end, the pandemic only underscored the urgent need to gather, to mourn, to begin to heal. Our communities have been decimated by violence and hard hit by this pandemic. In all too familiar ways, we are not counted, not visible.

I know now that this new coronavirus has forever changed us—but I do not want to go back. I hope that we have "hit rock bottom." The systems that make up the world that brought us to this point are not only dysfunctional, they are deadly. COVID-19 exposed and deepened the tragic realities that many of us confront every day. BIPOC, queer, and trans people will continue to fall victim to the systems of the old world, too often paying the price with our very lives. COVID-19 became an opportunity for a reset. I am hopeful that the emergence of the virus and the ensuing protests, boycotts, and signs of solidarity can and will carry us into a new world.

ABOUT THE AUTHOR

Michelle Veras identifies as Latina, mixed race, and queer. She has worked in the nonprofit sector for over twenty years. Her work has largely focused on the intersection of health, youth, and community development. Michelle received a Master of Public Health from Brown University in 2019. She is an activist and a mother living in Providence, Rhode Island, where she grew up. Michelle is projects director at the National LGBT Cancer Network.

NOTES

1   Steve Ahlquist, "Providence's First Annual People of Color Dyke and Trans March—Uprise RI," Uprise RI, June 16, 2019, accessed January 14, 2022, https://upriseri.com/2019-06-16-dtpoc.

QUEERS, COVID-19, AND MEDICARE FOR ALL
James McMaster

Queer activists were yelling at Pete Buttigieg again. This time it happened at a private fundraiser in San Francisco, Valentine's Day 2020. The time before that it was by a protestor at a fundraiser in Chicago. In both cases, the point the activists sought to make to the first gay candidate seriously considered for president of the United States was a simple one: you are too quick to abandon the most oppressed among us in exchange for upward mobility reserved only for yourself and those like you. Buttigieg, they insisted, was all assimilation and no liberation, not for queers, not for the Black folks of his hometown of South Bend, Indiana, not for anyone. So the activists, calling themselves #QueersAgainstPete, put forth their own vision for the world. Where Pete opposed universal free public college, the activists demanded it, where Pete supported an increase in military spending, the activists rejected it, and where Pete opposed the establishment of a universal single-payer health care system in the United States, the activists, quite rightly, insisted upon it.

This last critique brings me to the point of this essay. From the depths of the COVID-19 pandemic—as spring turned to summer, quarantined with my partner, working from home, managing emotions ranging from rage at my government to grief related to personal loss—I am writing to make the queer case for Medicare for All. It is clearer than ever that we must reject the mainstream moderation embodied by the Mayor

Petes of the world in pursuit of universal public goods, systems like Medicare for All, which guarantee all people tolerable lives regardless of their relationship to heteronormativity. By the end of this essay I hope you'll see why.

At this moment in history, thanks in large part to Senator Bernie Sanders and the movement at his back, the argument for Medicare for All is widely understood. The program, which would provide everyone in the United States, even noncitizens, with access to health care, would also eliminate co-pays, premiums, and deductibles and would do this while covering dental costs, mental health care costs, and the costs associated with reproductive health care, gender-affirming care, and the sort of long-term, at-home care needed by the disabled and elderly members of our communities. For these reasons, it should be no surprise that more than half of Americans polled support Medicare for All, which is good news for everyone, because, according to a Yale study,[1] the program would save the United States $450 billion in health care costs annually by eliminating administrative overhead and the profiteering of our totally incoherent private insurance industry.[2] The same study says that the policy would save sixty-eight thousand lives a year, the lives of people who would otherwise owe their deaths to being uninsured or underinsured. In 2018, according to census data, 27.5 million people were without health insurance.[3] To give you a sense of scale, that's millions more than the total number of people who live in New York State (19.45 million), a statistic that predates the first outbreak of COVID-19.

Again, in a post-pandemic world we need Medicare for All more than ever. In the first three months of the COVID-19 pandemic, over thirty million people filed for unemployment, and a great many of these people, who lost their jobs to the pandemic, lost their health care coverage with them.[4] In that same first three months of the pandemic, in the United States, more than seventy thousand people died of COVID-19, and those deaths were unevenly distributed along race and class lines.[5] According to an article published by the Intercept in early April 2020, "The death rate among Latino New Yorkers [was] 22.8 for every 100,000 people. Among African Americans, it [was] 19.8. In contrast, 10.2 of every 100,000 white New Yorkers [had] died from the new coronavirus."[6] I'm putting some focus on the empire state here, because Black and Brown New York City residents have been those most impacted by the coronavirus pandemic, partially because so many of them are the sort of workers without benefits whose heretofore undervalued labor has proven absolutely essential to the maintenance of our society in this time of crisis.

You will read these words long after I have finished writing them, and by that time all of these statistics—the death counts, the numbers of people unemployed and uninsured—will be much higher. Obviously, all of this will hit the marginalized hardest.

Queers, for example, many of them Black and Brown, are also especially vulnerable to COVID-19. In their open letter to South Bend's former mayor, written before the spread of COVID-19 across the United States, the #QueersAgainstPete organizers remind us that those who exist outside of cis- and heteronormativity, who are often cast out of their families of origin, are more likely to experience health care and housing insecurity.[7] Such persons, they argue, are, therefore, also more likely to be criminalized and incarcerated at much higher rates. We know now that incarcerated people, from Rikers Island to the concentration camps at the US southern border, have been some of the hardest hit by the pandemic. This is why queers across the country, whether working with Jewish Voice for Peace in New York City or the Party for Socialism and Liberation in Madison, Wisconsin, where I live, have dedicated themselves to the abolitionist efforts that have gathered under the digital rallying cry of #FreeThemAll. It matters, of course, that the #QueersAgainstPete letter was written and released prior to the worst days of COVID-19. This tells us something that everyone needs to know: the pandemic did not produce from scratch the social and economic ruptures that we now face; it merely exacerbated them. The problems that underpin our contemporary crises are old, structural, and due in large part to a mainstream ideology associated as much with Pete Buttigieg as it is with Donald Trump. Call this ideology *neoliberalism.*

Neoliberalism is a political, economic, and cultural philosophy that prioritizes markets and the profit motive above people and the public good.[8] It emerged in the United States under Ronald Reagan as a response, in part, to the liberation movements of the sixties and seventies. Economically, neoliberalism is associated with deregulation and privatization. Culturally, it is associated with the superficial inclusion and assimilation of marginalized peoples into pre-existing institutions rather than the interrogation and abolition of those institutions responsible for marginalizing people in the first place. While democratic socialists say that the state's responsibility is to care for its citizens, neoliberals say that it is the personal responsibility of the citizens to care for themselves, no matter what preexisting structures of domination make doing so difficult. While democratic socialists call for Medicare for All, neoliberals advance half measures. Obama's half-measure, even though he had the support of a democratic supermajority at the start of his first term, was the Affordable Care Act. Buttigieg's, of course, was Medicare for All Who Want It. It's the neoliberal thing to do to prioritize personal choice over universal access after all. I'm saying all of this to convince you of something: we must end the bipartisan neoliberal consensus—its moderation, its preference for profit over people, be they queer or not. This is what we have to blame for the massive premature death that we've seen both during and prior to the coronavirus pandemic.

Here's a real-life example. For most of my life, I didn't understand what health insurance was, because my family couldn't afford it. We would pay out of pocket when we went to the doctor or dentist, and so we tried to keep those visits to a minimum. (I now deal with chronic pain as a consequence.) I have memories of my dad complaining about Obamacare's individual mandate. He would say that some people who made too much money to qualify for government support were being fined for not buying insurance that they couldn't afford. So my single father, presumably one of these people, continued without health insurance, avoiding visits to the doctor until he couldn't any longer. Then, in 2014, a few days after Christmas, he died suddenly of a heart attack. He passed alone and in the middle of the night. He'd just turned sixty. I was twenty-four. I had to use GoFundMe to pay for his funeral. In a 2018 interview with CNN, Congresswoman Alexandria Ocasio-Cortez, perhaps drawing on what she learned from her own father's premature death, argued that death costs should be factored in as costs of the current health care system, and, as usual, she was right to do so. She would make a similar argument years later, after her district had already been deemed the nation's most ravaged by COVID-19. Her constituents were losing loved ones and, with them, to honor them, their livelihoods. When we talk about queer suffering in and after quarantine under our current health care system we must also talk about the costs queers must pay, emotionally and financially, when we lose our loved ones. Medicare for All would have saved my father's life, and, in many ways, my own. I know this for sure.

Another thing I know for sure is that my father was an American citizen, and were he not things would have been much worse. Many people come to the United States with papers but through no fault of their own end up undocumented. This means that even after living in the United States for three decades, even after all of the taxes they've paid since arriving in this country, the state sees no reason why it should provide them with access to health care. The fact is that undocumented immigrants in the United States struggle to receive employer-based insurance and are legally barred from Medicare, Medicaid, and the Affordable Care Act Marketplaces. While some are eventually able to access citizenship if sponsored by a blood relative or a spouse, others have neither blood relatives nor love interests in the United States to usher them into the exclusive club of citizenship.

Imagine for a moment what it must feel like to be undocumented in the midst of a global pandemic—to be deemed an "essential worker" but to know that if you get sick while performing that work the country you now call home will leave you to die. Imagine what it feels like to love an undocumented person like this—to not know when they were last seen by a doctor and to wonder what might have gone wrong since. Imagine the moments that will wash over you if you ever learn that your undocumented loved one, elderly and uninsured, has tested positive for COVID-19. Feel the dread that comes with the threat of loss as it mixes with the dread that comes with all the stupid questions you'll have to answer about cost, debt, and all the other hindrances to grief built into our current system.

Queer activism has long argued that human rights and material resources should not be reserved for those who fit neatly into the nuclear family or the couple form. People make loving lives in all sorts of social arrangements that exist outside of those recognized by the state as legitimate and deserving of government assistance. Such social arrangements are the stuff of queer kinship, whether they include queer-identified people or whether they look something more like a family of misfits, straight and not, who won't appear on paper, because they can't or won't replicate heteronormative mandates with the right amount of reverence. Queer activists seeking health care access must recognize that the radical potential of Medicare for All is not simply that it will provide all queer-identified persons with health care coverage. More than that, what makes Medicare for All so insurgent, so queer, is its promise to disentangle one's ability to access health care from one's ability to properly inhabit heteronormativity. Under Medicare for All, undocumented persons would be able to receive regular, life-sustaining care no matter how much money they make and no matter what their relationship to biological family and state-sanctioned romance. This, make no mistake, is revolutionary, and the political promise Medicare for All makes doesn't end there.

COVID-19 has precipitated the worst period of yellow peril anti-Asian racism I've known in my lifetime. I experienced self-quarantining as a relief from the possibility of harassment or assault, and I say this as a queer and mixed-race Filipino American who is only mistaken for Chinese by the most ignorant of passers-by. Of course, many Asian workers don't have the privilege to self-quarantine. These folks—care workers, grocery store workers, tipped workers, social workers, the houseless, etc.—are especially vulnerable to xenophobic violence, doubly so if they live in overwhelmingly white areas. As I've already established, Medicare for All is a race issue in many ways, and one of them is that this period of anti-Asian animus would be reduced in length and intensity if the United States were responding to this pandemic from the high ground of a single-payer health care system.

I'll conclude simply by saying that COVID-19 has exposed this country for what it is: both structured and ravaged by white settler supremacy, heteropatriarchy, and neoliberal capitalism. People, many whom we love, have fallen to their deaths through the holes of a barely existent US social safety net that these oppressive forces have eviscerated over many decades. Now, more than ever before in my lifetime, people are eager to rise up and demand what they deserve—not a government that insists that we each take personal responsibility for our malnourishment and premature death but a government whose raison d'être is to ensure that its people, including those who are undocumented and incarcerated, are cared for regardless of what might befall them. If we are all in this together, it is because we are interdependent beings. It is because we need one another, because we are only as strong as the most vulnerable among us. Queers, of course, learned these lessons decades ago while watching loved ones die of AIDS on Reagan's negligent, homophobic watch. Just as we argued then against that neoliberal regime for health care as a human right, we dismiss today anyone who tries to sell us a half measure, a false unity, or anything short of a queer socialist belief in universal public goods—be they the president or just a gay mayor who really wanted to be. We do this for one another, because it is what it will take to win the life-saving something that is Medicare for All. We do this, because it is what it will take to keep Medicare for All once we've won it. We do this, because the alternative is too dark, too callous, too painful to bear.

ABOUT THE AUTHOR

James McMaster is assistant professor of Gender and Women's Studies and Asian American Studies at University of Wisconsin-Madison. He is currently working on a book project that puts the discourse of care theory into conversation with queer, feminist, and Asian Americanist critique and cultural production. His writing has appeared in the *Journal of Asian American Studies*, *American Quarterly*, *TDR/The Drama Review*, *Transgender Studies Quarterly*, and *Women & Performance: a journal of feminist theory*, where he is also the coeditor, with Olivia Michiko Gagnon, of a special issue titled *The Between: Couple Forms, Performing Together*.

NOTES

1   Alison P. Galvani, Alyssa S. Parpia, Eric M. Foster, Burton H. Singer, and Meagan C. Fitzpatrick, "Improving the Prognosis of Health Care in the USA," *Lancet*, 395, no. 10223 (February 2020): 524–33.

2   Jason Lemon, "Support for Medicare for All in US Surges Amid Coronavirus Pandemic, New Poll Shows," *Newsweek*, April 1, 2020, accessed January 14, 2022, https://www.newsweek.com/support-medicare-all-us-surges-amid-coronavirus-pandemic-new-poll-shows-1495574.

3   Dylan Scott, "The Uninsured Rate Had Been Steadily Declining for a Decade. But Now It's Rising Again," Vox, September 10, 2019, accessed January 14, 2022, https://www.vox.com/policy-and-politics/2019/9/10/20858938/health-insurance-census-bureau-data-trump.

4   Christopher Rugaber, "30 Million Have Sought US Unemployment Aid Since Virus Hit," Associated Press, April 30, 2020, accessed January 14, 2021, https://apnews.com/7f38d7fa2982dc53572232c9d2049dca.

5   Reuters, "U.S. Coronavirus Deaths Exceed 70,000 as Forecasting Models Predict Grim Summer, *New York Times*, May 5, 2020, accessed January 14, 2022, https://www.nytimes.com/reuters/2020/05/05/us/05reuters-health-coronavirus-usa-casualties.html.

6   Sharon Lerner, "Coronavirus Numbers Reflect New York City's Deep Economic Divide," Intercept, April 9, 2020, accessed January 14, 2022, https://theintercept.com/2020/04/09/nyc-coronavirus-deaths-race-economic-divide.

7   "Open Letter," #QueersAgainstPete, accessed January 14, 2022, https://qapb.squarespace.com/letter.

8   For more detailed accounts of neoliberalism see Lisa Duggan, *The Twilight of Equality: Neoliberalism, Cultural Politics, and the Attack on Democracy* (Boston, MA: Beacon Press, 2003); Roderick Ferguson, *The Reorder of Things: The University and Its Pedagogies of Minority Difference* (Minneapolis: University of Minnesota Press, 2012); Grace Kyungyon Hong, *Death Beyond Disavowal: The Impossible Politics of Difference* (Minneapolis: Minnesota University Press, 2015); Jodi Melamed, *Represent and Destroy: Rationalizing Violence in the New Racial Capitalism* (Minneapolis: Minnesota University Press, 2011); Wendy Brown, *Undoing the Demos: Neoliberalism's Stealth Revolution* (New York: Zone Books, 2015).

SPIRALING INTO SELF-LOVE: THE WILDERNESS, THE JOURNEY, AND COVID-19

Mark Travis Rivera

"When it is dark, come back to self. When it is scary, come back to self. When it is hard, come back to self. When it is unknown, come back to self. When you are tired, come back to self. When you are hopeless, come back to self. When you are lost, come back to self."

—Joel Leon

I asked the Universe for love, and it gave me a mirror and said, "You are all the love you need."

If I am all the love I need, then why does it feel so excruciating, lonely, and painful?

In the eighth week of shelter-in-place in Oakland, California, I started musing on what the Universe had told me. The truth is that I am often seeking love and validation from others, because I struggle to accept my own innate worthiness. To be Latinx, disabled, gay, and femme is to live at the intersection of so many narratives that tell me I am not worthy.

After nearly a decade of therapy, I am realizing that my need to feel validated stems from the abandonment issues I dealt with as a child, my father having left my mother before I was even born. As I got older, being a bastard son really plagued me. It tainted all my interactions with other men and set me up for a race I would not be able to finish. What does a young gay person do when they are trying to fill a void? I turned to sex. Losing my virginity at the age of fourteen and living life quite recklessly—I realized that some men didn't mind using my body, and I desperately wanted to be held by a man's arms.

So what happens when a global pandemic breaks out and you are forced into self-isolation? For me, it was an opportunity to embrace myself. I faced the parts of myself that are hard to love and tried so desperately to meet myself with empathy, compassion, and grace. Prior to COVID-19, I thought I had a strong handle on my struggle with self-worth. I have been committed to doing the work in therapy. Then my daily routine was taken from me. If I am being honest, I used work and my routine to distract me from the inner-me that still struggles.

Dr. Brené Brown talks about staying so busy in our lives that we numb ourselves from feeling pain and sorrow and from facing the reality of our lives. I first discovered Dr. Brown's work in the summer of 2013 through Oprah's Super Soul Sunday, and I was instantly hooked. COVID-19 slapped me back to reality. There's no escaping that I am still hustling for my worthiness. Normally I would drink a glass or two of wine to be numb, but I made the decision to stop drinking a couple of weeks before the pandemic broke out. You're probably thinking, "What was he thinking, quitting drinking during this time?" You would be right to think that, but I had recognized that drinking was causing me more harm than good. As a person who has bipolar disorder and depression, drinking was a way to self-medicate, and it was destructive to my well-being. With three months sober and in quarantine, I became even more aware of my feelings and the need to be loved by someone else. Sobriety has been hard for me, because I have become too accustomed to drinking my problems away. After three months of sobriety during the pandemic, I had a relapse. A few drinks after a really rough day and I would normally spiral out of control with shame, but I knew that this journey toward sobriety, especially during a global pandemic, would have its setbacks.

While I was still a fetus in my mother's womb, my father left her. I would spend a lot of time yearning for fatherly love—the kind you see in movies and on television, where the father teaches his son how to play sports and how to be a man. As I explore inner-work, I acknowledge that the deeply rooted pain I have yet to recover from is my first experience with double abandonment, both mine and my mother's. For years, I would blame myself for my father leaving, but as I grew up I realized his inability to be a dad had nothing to do with me. He was just repeating the cycle he grew up with, and instead of being a better father than his own dad, he followed in those footsteps. Now I am learning that loving myself is the only way to fill the void my father created.

I wish I could write that this journey has been easy. I wish I could offer you steps to follow that will make loving yourself easier, but I can't. We are imperfect beings, and embracing those imperfections and loving ourselves despite them is the key to true freedom. To quote Dr. Brown from her book *Braving the Wilderness*, "True belonging is the spiritual practice of believing in and belonging to yourself so deeply that you can share your most authentic self with the world and find sacredness in both being a part of something and standing alone in the wilderness. True belonging doesn't require you to change who you are; it requires you to be who you are."

I am moving toward self-love by allowing myself to show myself grace and mercy. To think about all the ways I have survived this cruel world and still managed to be loving. To be loving and kind in a world that has tried to strip me of my humanity, of my own innate worthiness, just proves that self-love is neither a lofty idea that's become trendy nor egotistical; it's a means of survival in a world that claims you are not lovable. In a period of self-isolation, away from my friends and my lover, I learned and am still learning that loving myself is keeping me alive and allowing me to have hope for the world that will exist after COVID-19, that this new world will leave room for loving yourself unapologetically.

ABOUT THE AUTHOR

An award-winning activist, author, choreographer, speaker, and writer, **Mark Travis Rivera** creates artwork that reflects his lived experience as a Latinx, disabled, gay, and gender nonconforming artist. As a dancer, he has apprenticed for Heidi Latsky Dance (New York City) and AXIS Dance Company (Oakland, California). He earned a BA in women's and gender studies, with a minor in public relations, from William Paterson University. As an activist, he has spoken in front of audiences at Harvard University, New York University, and MIT, to name a few. As a writer, he has been published in the Huffington Post, Fox News Latino, and North Jersey Media Group. In August 2017, Rivera published his first collection of poems and essays, *Drafts: An Imperfect Collection of Writing*. To learn more, visit www.MarkTravisRivera.com.

FOUR THINGS WE MUST DO TO FIGHT MEDICAL MISTRUST AFTER THE COVID-19 PANDEMIC ENDS

Kenyon Farrow

In late 2020, the Centers for Disease Control and Prevention (CDC) made its recommendations for how best to distribute the two new COVID-19 vaccines that were expected to soon get Food and Drug Administration (FDA) emergency authorization approval. As anticipated, their recommendations focused on getting the vaccine first to health care workers and other frontline staff who had been caring for populations most at risk of illness and death from COVID-19, followed by senior citizens, people with comorbidities, such as heart disease and diabetes, and then down the line to everyone else.

Throughout the pandemic, there had been considerable reporting on the rise of vaccine skepticism on the part of the American public. Some of that reporting was focused on what role medical mistrust among Black people would mean for our willingness to get the vaccine once it became available, in light of the fact that Black people in America are far more likely than whites to contract COVID-19 and to die from it.

Trump's Health and Human Services (HHS) Secretary Alex Azar publicly said that the federal agency was preparing a public education campaign to explain how the vaccine worked, what it does in the body, and the process for getting vaccinated. I agree that we need such an educational campaign; for one, so as to not leave people reliant on the opinions of their favorite pop star or social media influencer for critical information regarding their health. But it's also true that public health experts and federal agencies must think beyond the COVID-19 crisis. We have to begin to reinvest and reimagine public health to empower more people to make decisions based on the best available evidence, not on rhetoric from anti-science religious zealots, right-wing populists, or even Black "natural" health gurus who think a vegan diet is the cure-all for infectious-disease pandemics.

Whatever the root causes, we have to figure it out. Trying to do so in the middle of the worst pandemic in a hundred years (which, in the end, may top the 1918 flu pandemic) is a terrible way to do public health. If we are to be in better shape to deal with the next pandemic, here are four key actions that need to be taken.

Invest in Research to Understand Medical Mistrust. . .

There are many levels to—and a complicated history behind— medical mistrust in America. Mistrust among Black folks can be traced back to the story of Henrietta Lacks or the Tuskegee Syphilis Study, among other horrific abuses and experiments. There are stories of forced sterilizations of Black, Indigenous, and Latinx people, people with disabilities, and sometimes even poor whites dating back to the early 1900s. There's also medical mistrust based on the present-day realities of being Black and trying to get quality health care without your concerns being ignored and without being condescended to by providers or administrative staff.

Then there are the conspiracy theories that go beyond mistrust. These speak to the belief that there is active malfeasance on behalf of governments or companies to engineer diseases to kill specific groups of people, that vaccines and therapeutics are developed to inject unsuspecting people with various tracking or surveillance devices, and that public health is rooted in creating pretexts for massive social control. Some of these phenomena are caused or exacerbated by historical truths, while some are caused by people wanting to center themselves as healers in pursuit of a quick buck. It's also the case for many people that being anti-establishment and anti–any established set of facts or truth, whether one is a leftist or a right-wing conservative, becomes a kind of identity, a badge of honor to set oneself apart from the pack.

While these are all distinct phenomena that sometimes overlap, it stands to reason that we have very little research on the biological, political, cultural, or social forces that explain medical mistrust. There is an urgent need for public health research portfolios at the National Institutes of Health (NIH), the CDC, and other research agencies to increase funding for studies aimed at better understanding the basis for medical mistrust and health-related conspiracy beliefs. This includes research on the relationship between social media and the proliferation of misinformation that helps promote conspiracy theories, junk science, and the apparent increasing distrust of established scientific processes and public health protocols.

. . . And Then Invest in Solutions to Address It!

In addition to researching medical mistrust and conspiracy theories, there is an urgent need for funding strategies dedicated to addressing the issues outlined above as regular and ongoing aspects of public health programs. The CDC, the Health Resources and Services Administration (HRSA), and other grantmaking public health agencies should be tasked with funding demonstration projects that are aimed at cultivating community-driven strategies to address public health, biomedical research, and health care–related mistrust, misinformation, and conspiracy theories.

Many of us who've worked in HIV prevention and care at the community level have had to create responses to theories that the government or pharmaceutical companies have a cure and are keeping it out of the reach of those who stand to benefit from it. Trying to explain to a layperson the role of the NIH, biotech vs. pharmaceutical companies, and regulatory agencies like the FDA is near impossible at a time when people are in a state of sheer terror about the COVID-19 crisis.

To my knowledge, there is currently no toolkit, training, or support that exists at the federal level to help frontline public health workers engage and address these issues as they arise. In the case of COVID-19, it may be that community-based HIV organizations are already best positioned to do this kind of work, given their relationships to other community institutions, where they often carry out prevention education, HIV testing, and linkage to care or pre-exposure prophylaxis (PrEP) services. But who offers this kind of training to the public health workforce? Is it taught in public health, nursing, or medical school programs?

Making science and public health institutions and regulatory bodies more transparent about their processes and teaching the history of medical racism, sexism, homophobia, and transphobia are essential to building and cultivating public trust. The CDC has to allow for (or perhaps hire) communications experts to develop new and novel approaches to break through to audiences, particularly those on social media. Often, the current messaging is frankly stodgy, boring, and not engaging enough to compete with the snark and quippy nature of social media communication styles.

Put Black Medical Providers, Researchers, and Policy Experts at the Center

One of the major reasons medical mistrust persists in Black communities in the US is that, despite the presence of Black medical doctors, researchers, and infectious-disease experts and activists, we are very rarely called upon by mainstream press or even social justice organizations to speak to the public about health-related issues (like COVID-19). I have personally complained to friends who run social justice organizations that were holding online events about racial disparities and COVID-19 that often featured no epidemiologists, researchers, medical providers, or public health activists who could offer the perspective needed to communicate the current medical research on COVID-19 and vaccination and help break through the mistrust.

It's not just government agencies that need to shift their thinking. Most racial justice–focused philanthropy in the US has largely focused on racial disparities in the criminal justice system, almost to the exclusion of everything else. So despite the numbers of Black people who die prematurely due to political and social forces that put us at very high risk of illness and disease and the persisting racism in health systems that means we often receive low-quality health care, there are very few funders who are willing to support the organizing, base building, and political-education campaigns to empower Black communities to fight on these fronts. In other words, Black Lives Matter, and not just when we die at the end of a police revolver.

Many racial justice funders were generous in moving money to organizations in need of COVID-19 relief for their workers or staff, but many of these funders were totally absent from supporting grassroots, community-based organizing efforts urging more accountability from health care systems, public health, and biomedical research. This work was mostly left to the most underfunded, scrappy conglomeration of Black activists doing work around drug policy and harm reduction, HIV, disability, and reproductive justice, who rely on a small handful of dedicated funders. Funders should be looking in the mirror and asking themselves why the anti-mask/anti-vaxxer white nationalist groups have out-mobilized the left on public health to the extent that governments are curbing smart public health strategies to appease these groups.

Start Making Changes in the Public Health Sector

Lastly, public health is due for its own reckoning. Like most institutions in the US, it still suffers from white paternalism, is obsessed with behavior-change strategies (over and above systemic forces that shape the health-related decisions people are actually empowered to make), and still operates in a way that resembles aspects of our policing and carceral systems. For example, epidemiology still refers to its efforts to track health conditions as "surveillance." HIV and disability justice activists have probably been the most vocal about pushing public health authorities to use "people first" language and to stop referring to people as "infected," "spreaders," "defaulters," or "noncompliant."

We not only have to reinvent the language we use, but we have to be willing to reimagine strategies around contact tracing and partner notification. The current strategies have resulted in people being fearful of engaging public health entities, especially when biometric companies are already positioning themselves as the solution to getting out of lockdown, offering many more ways for people's human rights to be violated and for data to be collected by unaccountable profiteers.

Instead, we should more readily bring the kind of bioethics frameworks and protocols that exist in biomedical research into public health practice. Doing so would be a useful tool to help shift public health institutions into thinking more critically about how their practices do or do not align with a human rights approach.

As a public health community, we have a lot of work to do. We will roll out vaccines, and I think most people will eventually take them. While COVID-19 may become a disease of the past, we can't rest on our laurels. We have to do the ongoing work to transform the role of public health and make it visible and something people can relate to, and Black public health practitioners have to play a leading role, especially where our communities are impacted.

I'm hoping new leadership in the federal agencies will make this possible. I am also hoping my fellow social justice warriors who have long ignored HIV and other public health issues will continue to see us as allies in the work of building the world and society that we all want to, and can, live and thrive in.

ABOUT THE AUTHOR

Kenyon Farrow was the senior editor of TheBody/TheBodyPro from 2017 to 2020. He is the co-executive director of Partners for Dignity & Rights, a US organization advocating for social and systemic justice. This chapter was originally published on TheBodyPro, which informs and supports people whose work intersects with the HIV/AIDS epidemic. We have republished it with their permission.

MACHO, MACHO MAN: WHAT WE LEARNED ABOUT MASCULINITY FROM COVID-19

Peter Frycki

During the COVID-19 pandemic we learned that men were more skeptical than women about COVID-19 vaccines and wearing masks, but the real divide that threatened a "new normal" and the opportunity to reopen post pandemic was between men who were trying to project masculinity and the men who weren't. Men who asserted a traditionally masculine gender identity were less likely to say that they would get the COVID-19 vaccine, according to a 2021 study by researchers at Fairleigh Dickinson University.[1]

The data demonstrated that more masculine men were likely to say that a vaccine may have side effects and were more resistant to wearing masks for protection. They were also more likely to say they have been diagnosed with COVID-19.

"Men's attempts to demonstrate what they believe to be masculine behavior may be holding back the country's response to the COVID-19 pandemic," said Dan Cassino, a professor at Fairleigh Dickinson University who studies masculinity and is the director of the poll. "Many men think that being tough is part of being masculine. That means not wearing a mask, or getting a vaccine. It means they figure they'll be tough enough to survive COVID anyway."

Resistance to measures designed to limit the spread of a dangerous virus left these men at greater risk of contracting it. Men who asserted a "completely masculine" gender were more likely to report having been diagnosed with the COVID-19 virus. For example, 2.2 percent of "completely masculine" men say that they were diagnosed with COVID-19, compared with 0.8 percent of other men. About 1.4 percent of women, across gender categories, say that they were diagnosed with the virus in the same time period.

Although the difference was rather small, the large sample size of the survey and the closeness of the figures to zero means that the difference is well within the normal range of statistical significance, given a sample of over six thousand respondents. Some individuals reported being unsure if they had been diagnosed or not and were excluded from the analysis. If those individuals were included, 2.2 percent of "completely masculine" men say that they were diagnosed, compared with 0.7 percent of other men. This figure also does not include individuals who may have been infected but didn't see a medical professional.

Put another way, men who were trying to assert their masculinity were just shy of three times as likely to report having been diagnosed with COVID-19. The results are not a problem of men bragging or over-reporting, says Cassino. "If anything, we'd guess that men concerned with their masculinity are less likely to see a doctor, so this is a real difference, rather than just a difference in reporting," said Cassino. "We can't exclude the possibility that men are over-reporting having been diagnosed, but the results line up with all of the reported high-risk behaviors in this group. Trying to be macho has real consequences for some men."

Respondents in the study were asked to place their gender identity on a six-point scale from "completely masculine" to "completely feminine." About two-thirds of US men (68 percent) placed themselves as "completely masculine," compared with 57 percent of women who said that they are "completely feminine."

Only about four percent of men say that they're "feminine," while eight percent of women called themselves "masculine." Past research has shown this to be strongly related to age and religious views among men.[2]

Those men who asserted "complete masculinity" were more likely than other men to express skepticism about coronavirus vaccines and were less likely to say that they would take the vaccine. Thus, 21 percent of men who asserted a "completely masculine" gender identity say that they were "very unlikely" to get a coronavirus vaccination when it became available to them, compared with 17 percent of other men. Another key issue is that this group was three times more likely to get COVID-19.

"The idea here is that if you're strong enough, you don't need to take vaccines," said Cassino. "For these men, saying that you don't want to take preventative measures is a way of showing strength."

Justifying reluctance to get the vaccine means that "masculine" men were more likely to say that vaccines are actually a bad thing. "On average, men who insist on a 'completely masculine gender identity say that there's a 22 percent chance that the vaccine will cause serious side effects, compared with 19 percent of other men. It's no surprise, then, that 34 percent of them agreed with a statement that COVID-19 vaccines have many harmful known side effects, compared to 27 percent of other men."

Reticence to embrace measures intended to limit the spread of COVID-19 extends past vaccine skepticism. Ten percent of "completely masculine" men said wearing a face mask was dangerous to the health of the wearer, compared to just 6 percent of other men. Seventeen percent of those men agreed that masks are too uncomfortable to wear, compared with 13 percent of other men. They were also resistant to the idea that they could be forced to wear a mask: 24 percent of them agreed with the statement, "We live in a free country, and no one can force me to wear a mask," compared with 17 percent of other men, and 18 percent of the overall population.

"Refusing to wear a mask is a public way for men to show how tough they are," said Cassino. "Unlike a vaccine, the absent mask is a visible symbol of your beliefs, a way to signal to everyone around you that you don't need to take preventative measures."

The same factors that led men to avoid masks in an attempt to assert their masculinity also led them to ignore other COVID-19 mitigation behaviors recommended by public health authorities. Forty-three percent of "completely masculine" men say that they had visitors at their residence, compared with 36 percent of other men. Sixteen percent say that they attended a gathering of ten or more people, compared with 10 percent of other men and 11 percent of the overall population.

What does all of this mean for the future? The COVID-19 pandemic clarified the intersections between "completely masculine" identities and public health. How we as a population choose to implement these lessons as we move beyond COVID-19 is perhaps the question public health experts and gender studies scholars will continue to grapple with.

The analysis described here relies on data from surveys administered by the Understanding America Study (https://uasdata.usc.edu/index.php), which is maintained by the Center for Economic and Social Research at the University of Southern California. The Fairleigh Dickinson University Poll questions were included in the survey. Results are based on a sample size of 6,179, surveyed between January 6 and February 1, 2021.

This article was originally published by *Out in Jersey* on February 21, 2021, and is reprinted with permission.

ABOUT THE AUTHOR
Peter Frycki is the publisher of *Out in Jersey* magazine and an occasional writer. His previous occupations were with the Mercer County Board of Social Services in Trenton as a caseworker and supervisor.

NOTES
1   "FDU Poll Finds Masculinity Is a Major Risk Factor for COVID-19," Fairleigh Dickinson University Poll, February 16, 2021, accessed January 17, 2022, https://www.fdu.edu/news/fdu-poll-finds-masculinity-is-a-major-risk-factor-for-covid-19; all Dan Cassino quotes in this chapter come from this document.

2   Dan Cassino, "Moving Beyond Sex: Measuring Gender Identity in Telephone Surveys," *Survey Practice* 13, no. 1, accessed January 17, 2022, https://tinyurl.com/37jkd2th.

REOPENING THE PAST OR REIMAGINING THE FUTURE?
Adrian Shanker

Rabbi Morgan Forrest, a queer, Jewish, disabled study partner of mine shared: "The one thing COVID-19 brought me was this period of time when the doors of online connections are wide open. I fear that once everyone goes back to their usual and customary pre-COVID routines, those of us who are disabled, health-challenged, or home-bound will once again be forgotten and left behind."

There's no contemporary roadmap for what happens after a pandemic. Does a light switch flip and everything returns to pre-pandemic times? Is that even possible? Is that a good thing even if it were possible? What do we say to those who have found solace, community, and connectivity in the virtual world that COVID-19 necessitated? To be sure, the social isolation of the first year of the COVID-19 pandemic was not easy on anyone. Early in the pandemic, people joked that introverts had been preparing for it their whole lives, but with what felt like no end in sight, the mental health considerations of prolonged social isolation began to increase. However, our communities did transition quickly to create virtual programs, online communities, and connections across time and space. We radically reimagined communities to create connectivity in the cloud. This was our COVID-19 resiliency, and there is no reason for it to end as the world reopens.

Even as I longed for the return of in-person connections, travel, and gatherings of friends and family, all of which were precluded by the pandemic before the approval of COVID-19 vaccines, I hated to hear people longing for a return to normal. Fuck normal. Pre-COVID normal wasn't working for anyone.

What does "fuck normal" mean? And why isn't returning to the past the best outcome? After all, isn't that what the whole world is waiting for? Pre-COVID normal was inflexible and competitive. The pandemic required mutual aid and an abundance of community care. Pre-COVID normal was capitalistic and punitive. The pandemic required activists to call for an end to evictions and the release of incarcerated people from crowded prisons. So, yes, with the reopening of much of our society after many people could access COVID-19 vaccines, the human desire to hug each other again was palpable. But instead of simply reopening the past, we have an opportunity to reimagine the future based not on what we once knew existed but instead on what we now know to be possible.

In *When Brooklyn Was Queer*, historian Hugh Ryan writes, "I look forward to a future where we also have a past." When engaging in the creative and radical act of reimagining, we can remember both what worked and what didn't work before and during the COVID-19 pandemic. We can imagine a future where access to community can be bridged across geography and ability. A future where instead of prisons or police, we invest in community-driven models for accountability and restorative justice. We can learn from the vaccine distribution efforts and imagine a future where we always consider people with underlying health conditions first. We can learn from mutual aid networks to imagine a future where we all take care of each other. The individualization of the normal from pre-pandemic times may not work for us as we move forward. The COVID-19 pandemic has reminded us that all we really have is, in fact, each other.

Likewise, the COVID-19 pandemic did not create the disparities that left BIPOC, queer, and disabled communities behind, these disparities have long existed. The COVID-19 pandemic made them worse. But throughout the pandemic, queer activists responded with care for each other and our community. Queer organizations found that through virtual program offerings, they could reach community members who were never able to participate previously when access considerations were not considered. As the broader society learned that reopening with an equity lens requires centering the needs of historically excluded and minoritized populations, queer organizations were reminded of this as well. Many queer organizations reopened with hybrid technology that maintained community connectivity for disabled community members. A reimagined future empowers us to rebuild from the margins.

COVID-19 taught us that the greatest threats to our society might or might not be a virus that none of us can see. It might be the parts of "normal" that we had grown accustomed to before the pandemic and that we have learned we do not want to take with us into the future. COVID-19 was traumatic and deadly. There is no silver lining to such a dangerous virus. But throughout the COVID-19 pandemic, we learned to care for each other in new and creative ways. We learned that in a reimagined future, we don't have to leave anyone behind. We learned how to respond to a crisis with care.

CONCLUSION
Adrian Shanker

Other books will surely detail the epidemiological failures that enabled COVID-19 to wreak such terrible damage on our communities. This book sought to present a different story: how queer activists responded to a crisis with care, compassion, resiliency, and results.

The COVID-19 pandemic taught us how much we rely on essential workers: delivery workers, health care workers, grocery store workers, and others—so after COVID-19, we should treat these workers like heroes every day, not only when we need to put their bodies on the line.

The COVID-19 pandemic taught us how important universal health care is: access to COVID-19 testing, treatment, and vaccinations were free for those without insurance—so after COVID-19, we should fight for a Medicare for All system, because health care is a human right, and our bodies deserve access to care at all stages of our lives.

The COVID-19 pandemic taught us that prisons are a cruel and unusual punishment; they are literal petri dishes where physical distancing is impossible and hand sanitizer is contraband—so after COVID-19 we should fight to abolish unjust systems and create community-based models of accountability and restorative justice.

The COVID-19 pandemic taught us that drastic changes are possible: schools were closed, businesses were shut down, and even the US federal tax deadline was moved—so after

COVID-19, activists should demand the big structural changes our communities need. We can no longer pretend that change is impossible.

We learned a great deal about how our society can be improved because of the COVID-19 pandemic. Now it's up to every one of us to radically reimagine our society so that the care and compassion we learned during the COVID-19 pandemic can be incorporated into all aspects of our lives.

ACKNOWLEDGMENTS

This text is written with gratitude for community and resiliency in uncertain times.

Thank you to the contributing authors: Sigfried Aragona, Kenyon Farrow, Peter Frycki, Jamie Gliksberg, Omar Gonzalez-Pagan, James McMaster, Emmett Patterson, Mark Travis Rivera, Denise Spivak, Michelle Veras, and Zephyr Williams. Special gratitude for Rea Carey for writing the foreword to this book.

Thank you to the entire team at PM Press, especially Steven Stothard, Stephanie Pasvankias, and Michael Ryan, and to John Yates of Stealworks for designing the book cover and briandesign for the interior book design.

Finally, thank you to the queer activists everywhere who relentlessly advocated, created, and imagined equity, access, and possibility during the COVID-19 pandemic. May we all take these lessons into the future and create the reimagined communities queer people deserve!

≡

ABOUT THE AUTHORS

Adrian Shanker (he/him) is editor of the critically acclaimed anthology *Bodies and Barriers: Queer Activists on Health* (PM Press, 2020) and the executive director of the Spahr Center, serving Marin County, California's LGBTQ+ and HIV communities. He previously founded and led Bradbury-Sullivan LGBT Community Center in Allentown, Pennsylvania. A specialist in LGBTQ+ health policy, he has developed leading-edge health promotion campaigns to advance health equity through behavioral, clinical, and policy changes. Adrian is also a member of the Presidential Advisory Council on HIV/AIDS.

Rea Carey served as the National LGBTQ Task Force's executive director from 2008 to 2021 and has advanced a vision of freedom for LGBTQ+ people and their families that is broad, inclusive, and progressive. She grounds her work solidly in racial, economic, gender, and social justice. Currently, Rea is the principal of Carey Forward consulting, providing executive coaching and working with executives and boards to provide strategic advice, succession and transition planning, crisis management, and to sharpen their leadership skills. Carey is a Hunt Alternatives' Prime Movers Fellow and serves on the boards of directors of the Flamboyan Foundation and the Freeman Foundation.

ABOUT PM PRESS

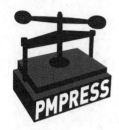

PM Press is an independent, radical publisher of books and media to educate, entertain, and inspire. Founded in 2007 by a small group of people with decades of publishing, media, and organizing experience, PM Press amplifies the voices of radical authors, artists, and activists. Our aim is to deliver bold political ideas and vital stories to all walks of life and arm the dreamers to demand the impossible. We have sold millions of copies of our books, most often one at a time, face to face. We're old enough to know what we're doing and young enough to know what's at stake. Join us to create a better world.

PM Press
PO Box 23912
Oakland, CA 94623
www.pmpress.org

PM Press in Europe
europe@pmpress.org
www.pmpress.org.uk

FRIENDS OF PM PRESS

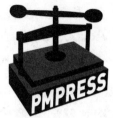

These are indisputably momentous times—the financial system is melting down globally and the Empire is stumbling. Now more than ever there is a vital need for radical ideas.

In the many years since its founding—and on a mere shoestring—PM Press has risen to the formidable challenge of publishing and distributing knowledge and entertainment for the struggles ahead. With hundreds of releases to date, we have published an impressive and stimulating array of literature, art, music, politics, and culture. Using every available medium, we've succeeded in connecting those hungry for ideas and information to those putting them into practice.

Friends of PM allows you to directly help impact, amplify, and revitalize the discourse and actions of radical writers, filmmakers, and artists. It provides us with a stable foundation from which we can build upon our early successes and provides a much-needed subsidy for the materials that can't necessarily pay their own way. You can help make that happen—and receive every new title automatically delivered to your door once a month—by joining as a Friend of PM Press. And, we'll throw in a free T-shirt when you sign up.

Here are your options:

- **$30 a month** Get all books and pamphlets plus 50% discount on all webstore purchases

- **$40 a month** Get all PM Press releases (including CDs and DVDs) plus 50% discount on all webstore purchases

- **$100 a month** Superstar—Everything plus PM merchandise, free downloads, and 50% discount on all webstore purchases

For those who can't afford $30 or more a month, we have **Sustainer Rates** at $15, $10 and $5. Sustainers get a free PM Press T-shirt and a 50% discount on all purchases from our website.

Your Visa or Mastercard will be billed once a month, until you tell us to stop. Or until our efforts succeed in bringing the revolution around. Or the financial meltdown of Capital makes plastic redundant. Whichever comes first.

Bodies and Barriers: Queer Activists on Health

Adrian Shanker with a Foreword
by Rachel L. Levine, MD and an
Afterword by Kate Kendell

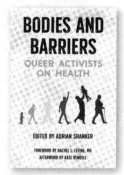

ISBN: 978-1-62963-784-6
$20.00   256 pages

LGBT people pervasively experience health
disparities, affecting every part of their bodies
and lives. Yet many are still grappling to understand the mutually
reinforcing health care challenges that lead to worsened health
outcomes. *Bodies and Barriers* informs health care professionals, students
in health professions, policymakers, and fellow activists about these
challenges, providing insights and a road map for action that could
improve queer health.

Through artfully articulated, data-informed essays by twenty-six well-
known and emerging queer activists—including Alisa Bowman, Jack
Harrison-Quintana, Liz Margolies, Robyn Ochs, Sean Strub, Justin Sabia-
Tanis, Ryan Thoreson, Imani Woody, and more—*Bodies and Barriers*
illuminates the health challenges LGBT people experience throughout
their lives and challenges conventional wisdom about health care
delivery. It probes deeply into the roots of the disparities faced by those
in the LGBT community and provides crucial information to fight for
health equity and better health outcomes.

The contributors to *Bodies and Barriers* look for tangible improvements,
drawing from the history of HIV/AIDS in the U.S. and from struggles
against health care bias and discrimination. At a galvanizing moment
when LGBT people have experienced great strides in lived equality, but
our health as a community still lags, here is an indispensable blueprint
for change by some of the most passionate and important health
activists in the LGBT movement today.

"Now, more than ever, we need Bodies and Barriers *to shine a spotlight on
how and why good healthcare for LGBTQ people and our families is such a
challenge.* Bodies and Barriers *provides a road map for all who are ready to
fight for health equity—in the doctor's office, in the halls of government, or
in the streets."*
—Rea Carey, executive director, National LGBTQ Task Force

Health Care Revolt: How to Organize, Build a Health Care System, and Resuscitate Democracy—All at the Same Time

Michael Fine
with a Foreword by Bernard Lown
and Ariel Lown Lewiton

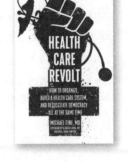

ISBN: 978-1-62963-581-1
$15.95   192 pages

The U.S. does not have a health system. Instead we have market for health-related goods and services, a market in which the few profit from the public's ill-health.

Health Care Revolt looks around the world for examples of health care systems that are effective and affordable, pictures such a system for the U.S., and creates a practical playbook for a political revolution in health care that will allow the nation to protect health while strengthening democracy.

Dr. Fine writes with the wisdom of a clinician, the savvy of a state public health commissioner, the precision of a scholar, and the energy and commitment of a community organizer.

"This is a revolutionary book. The author incites readers to embark on an audacious revolution to convert the American medical market into the American health care system."
—T.P. Gariepy, Stonehill College/CHOICE connect

"Michael Fine is one of the true heroes of primary care over several decades."
—Dr. Doug Henley, CEO and executive vice president of the American Academy of Family Physicians

"As Rhode Island's director of health, Dr. Fine brought a vision of a humane, local, integrated health care system that focused as much on health as on disease and treatment."
—U.S. Senator Sheldon Whitehouse

"Michael Fine has given us an extraordinary biopic on health care in America based on the authority of his forty-year career as writer, community organizer, family physician, and public health official."
—Fitzhugh Mullan, MD

Y'all Means All: The Emerging Voices Queering Appalachia

Edited by Z. Zane McNeill

ISBN: 978-1-62963-914-7
$20.00   200 pages

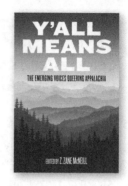

Y'all Means All is a celebration of the weird and wonderful aspects of a troubled region in all of their manifest glory! This collection is a thought-provoking hoot and a holler of "we're queer and we're here to stay, cause we're every bit a piece of the landscape as the rocks and the trees" echoing through the hills of Appalachia and into the boardrooms of every media outlet and opportunistic author seeking to define Appalachia from the outside for their own political agendas. Multidisciplinary and multi-genre, Y'all necessarily incorporates elements of critical theory, such as critical race theory and queer theory, while dealing with a multitude of methodologies, from quantitative analysis, to oral history and autoethnography.

This collection eschews the contemporary trend of "reactive" or "responsive" writing in the genre of Appalachian studies, and alternatively, provides examples of how modern Appalachians are defining themselves on their own terms. As such, it also serves as a toolkit for other Appalachian readers to follow suit, and similarly challenge the labels, stereotypes and definitions often thrust upon them. While providing blunt commentary on the region's past and present, the book's soul is sustained by the resilience, ingenuity, and spirit exhibited by the authors; values which have historically characterized the Appalachian region and are continuing to define its culture to the present.

This book demonstrates above all else that Appalachia and its people are filled with a vitality and passion for their region which will slowly but surely effect long-lasting and positive changes in the region. If historically Appalachia has been treated as a "mirror" of the country, this book breaks that trend by allowing modern Appalachians to examine their own reflections and to share their insights in an honest, unfiltered manner with the world.

Queercore: How to Punk a Revolution: An Oral History

Edited by Liam Warfield, Walter Crasshole, and Yony Leyser with an Introduction by Anna Joy Springer and Lynn Breedlove

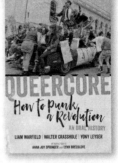

ISBN: 978-1-62963-796-9
$18.00   208 pages

Queercore: How to Punk a Revolution: An Oral History is the very first comprehensive overview of a movement that defied both the music underground and the LGBT mainstream community.

Through exclusive interviews with protagonists like Bruce LaBruce, G.B. Jones, Jayne County, Kathleen Hanna of Bikini Kill and Le Tigre, film director and author John Waters, Lynn Breedlove of Tribe 8, Jon Ginoli of Pansy Division, and many more, alongside a treasure trove of never-before-seen photographs and reprinted zines from the time, *Queercore* traces the history of a scene originally "fabricated" in the bedrooms and coffee shops of Toronto and San Francisco by a few young, queer punks to its emergence as a relevant and real revolution. *Queercore* is a down-to-details firsthand account of the movement explored by the people that lived it—from punk's early queer elements, to the moment that Toronto kids decided they needed to create a scene that didn't exist, to Pansy Division's infiltration of the mainstream, and the emergence of riot grrrl—as well as the clothes, zines, art, film, and music that made this movement an exciting middle finger to complacent gay and straight society. *Queercore* will stand as both a testament to radically gay politics and culture and an important reference for those who wish to better understand this explosive movement.

"*Finally, a book that centers on the wild, innovative, and fearless contributions queers made to punk rock, creating a punker-than-punk subculture beneath the subculture,* Queercore. *Gossipy and inspiring, a historical document and a call to arms during a time when the entire planet could use a dose of queer, creative rage.*"
—Michelle Tea, author of *Valencia*

"*I knew at an early age I didn't want to be part of a church, I wanted to be part of a circus. It's documents such as this book that give hope for our future. Anarchists, the queer community, the roots of punk, the Situationists, and all the other influential artistic guts eventually had to intersect.* Queercore *is completely logical, relevant, and badass.*"
—Justin Pearson, The Locust, Three One G

Facebooking the Anthropocene in Raja Ampat: Technics and Civilization in the 21st Century

Bob Ostertag

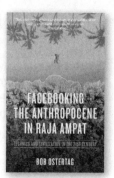

ISBN: 978-1-62963-830-0
$17.00   192 pages

The three essays of *Facebooking the Anthropocene in Raja Ampat* paint a deeply intimate portrait of the cataclysmic shifts between humans, technology, and the so-called natural world. Amid the breakneck pace of both technological advance and environmental collapse, Bob Ostertag explores how we are changing as fast as the world around us—from how we make music, to how we have sex, to what we do to survive, and who we imagine ourselves to be. And though the environmental crisis terrifies and technology overwhelms, Ostertag finds enough creativity, compassion, and humor in our evolving behavior to keep us laughing and inspired as the world we are building overtakes the world we found.

A true polymath who covered the wars in Central America during the 1980s, recorded dozens of music projects, and published books on startlingly eclectic subjects, Ostertag fuses his travels as a touring musician with his journalist's eye for detail and the long view of a historian. Wander both the physical and the intellectual world with him. Watch Buddhist monks take selfies while meditating and DJs who make millions of dollars pretend to turn knobs in front of crowds of thousands. Shiver with families huddling through the stinging Detroit winter without heat or electricity. Meet Spice Islanders who have never seen flushing toilets yet have gay hookup apps on their phones.

Our best writers have struggled with how to address the catastrophes of our time without looking away. Ostertag succeeds where others have failed, with the moral acuity of Susan Sontag, the technological savvy of Lewis Mumford, and the biting humor of Jonathan Swift.

"With deep intelligence and an acute and off-center sensibility, Robert Ostertag gives us a riveting and highly personalized view of globalization, from the soaring skyscapes of Shanghai to the darkened alleys of Yogyakarta."
—Frances Fox Piven, coauthor of *Regulating the Poor* and *Poor People's Movements*